Ayurvedic Kitchen Secrets

Balancing Body and Mind Through Ancient Recipes

Priya Anand

© Copyright 2024 - All rights reserved.

The content contained within this book may not be reproduced, duplicated or transmitted without direct written permission from the author or the publisher.

Under no circumstances will any blame or legal responsibility be held against the publisher, or author, for any damages, reparation, or monetary loss due to the information contained within this book, either directly or indirectly.

Legal Notice:

This book is copyright protected. It is only for personal use. You cannot amend, distribute, sell, use, quote or paraphrase any part, or the content within this book, without the consent of the author or publisher.

Disclaimer Notice:

Please note the information contained within this document is for educational and entertainment purposes only. All effort has been executed to present accurate, up to date, reliable, complete information. No warranties of any kind are declared or implied. Readers acknowledge that the author is not engaging in the rendering of legal, financial, medical or professional advice. The content within this book has been derived from various sources. Please consult a licensed professional before attempting any techniques outlined in this book.

By reading this document, the reader agrees that under no circumstances is the author responsible for any losses, direct or indirect, that are incurred as a result of the use of information contained within this document, including, but not limited to, errors, omissions, or inaccuracies.

Table of Contents

INTRODUCTION 5

CHAPTER I. Understanding Ayurveda 6

    Characteristics of each dosha 6

    How to identify your primary dosha 11

    Imbalances and their effects on health 18

CHAPTER II. The Ayurvedic Approach to Nutrition 23

    Food as medicine 23

    Importance of digestion and Agni (digestive fire) 29

    Six tastes (sweet, sour, salty, bitter, pungent, astringent) and their effects 33

    Eating according to your dosha 38

    Seasonal eating and its benefits 43

CHAPTER III. Ayurvedic Kitchen Essentials 48

    Common Ayurvedic spices and their healing properties 48

    Staple ingredients in an Ayurvedic kitchen 53

    Basic Ayurvedic cooking techniques (e.g., tempering spices, making ghee) 57

CHAPTER IV. Recipes for Vata Balance 62

    Warm porridges and nourishing smoothies 62

    Grounding soups and stews 66

    Hearty grains and root vegetables 71

Herbal teas and snacks to soothe Vata 77

CHAPTER V. Mindful Eating Practices 84

Setting up your dining space 84

The role of gratitude and mindfulness in eating 90

Pre-meal rituals 96

The importance of eating carefully 102

Gentle detox recipes and practices 106

CONCLUSION 113

INTRODUCTION

In "Ayurvedic Kitchen Secrets: Balancing Body and Mind Through Ancient Recipes," the culinary arts are used to bring the ageless wisdom of Ayurveda to life. This book explores the traditional Indian holistic health system and provides a wealth of recipes that support well-being and harmony. The "science of life," Ayurveda, places a strong emphasis on maintaining balance between the body, mind, and spirit. Our unique constitution, or dosha, may be balanced by matching our food to get optimum health and vigor.

The book serves as a guide to comprehending the fundamentals of Ayurvedic nutrition rather than merely being a compilation of recipes. The readers will learn how to determine their dosha and which meals are most appropriate for their individual requirements. Every dish is designed to improve general well-being, strengthen immunity, and aid with digestion. Invigorating vegetable dishes, healing spices, and calming teas and soups are just a few of the culinary adventures that "Ayurvedic Kitchen Secrets" offers.

The book simplifies the process of implementing Ayurvedic principles in daily life by emphasizing the use of seasonal, fresh products and straightforward preparation techniques. Regardless of your level of experience with Ayurveda, this book provides insightful analysis and useful advice to help you maximize the therapeutic benefits of food. Accept the age-old wisdom of Ayurveda and turn your kitchen into a happy and healthy haven.

CHAPTER I

Understanding Ayurveda

Characteristics of each dosha

Comprehending the doshas is essential to comprehending the human body and mind in Ayurvedic medicine, an age-old health and wellness philosophy that originated in India. The bio-energetic energies known as doshas control an individual's bodily and mental functions. The Vata, Pitta, and Kapha doshas are the three main types. The five elements are space, air, fire, water, and earth, and each dosha is made up of two of these elements. Each dosha has unique qualities that affect personality traits, physiological processes, and susceptibilities to different illnesses. The features of each dosha will be thoroughly examined in this section, offering readers a thorough grasp of their distinctive traits and how they appear in different people.

Vata dosha represents lightness, dryness, movement, and subtlety and is connected to the elements of air and space. People with mostly Vata dosha frequently have slender, fragile bodies, rough, dry skin, and a propensity for chilly extremities. They frequently follow strange eating and sleeping schedules and may have erratic energy levels. Vata's personalities are characterized by their fast thinking, enthusiasm, and adaptability. However, their mental activity can also cause worry, restlessness, and difficulty focusing.

The body's communication and mobility are governed by vata. Breathing, circulation, excretion, and nerve impulse transmission are all regulated by it. People who have a balanced Vata have great creativity and flexibility, as well as vigor and clear thinking. On the other hand, constipation, bloating, dry skin, sleeplessness, and anxiety are examples of physical and mental disorders that can arise from an imbalance in Vata. Vata types need to create routines, eat warm, nutritious foods, and practice soothing activities like yoga and meditation in order to stay in balance.

The fire and water aspects of the pitta dosha are represented by the attributes of heat, sharpness, intensity, and fluidity. Predominantly Pitta dosha individuals usually have a medium frame, well-defined muscles, warm skin, and a tendency to perspire readily. They frequently experience frequent feelings of hunger and thirst since they have a strong appetite and digestive system. Pitta personalities are renowned for their keen intelligence, tenacity, and capacity for leadership. They frequently have high goals, fierce competition, and intense love for what they do.

The body's metabolism and transformation are governed by the pita. It is in charge of energy generation, absorption, and digestion. Pitta also affects emotional equilibrium, skin tone, and eyesight. People with a balanced Pitta have clear skin, excellent digestion, and a keen mind. They possess the abilityto make well-informed judgments and stay focused on their goals. However, problems like rashes, irritation, wrath, acid reflux, and inflammation can result from an imbalance in Pitta. In order to stay in balance, Pitta types should steer clear of extremely hot and spicy meals, include foods that are cooling and hydrating in their diet, and learn stress-reduction practices.

The characteristics of weight, stability, dampness, and solidity are embodied by the kapha dosha, which is connected to the elements of earth and water. People with a strong Kapha dosha tend to be well-built, have shiny, smooth skin, and have a steady, composed manner. They frequently acquire weight and have slower metabolisms.

People who are kapha types are noted to be patient, kind, and caring. They frequently exhibit loyalty, dependability, and a high degree of endurance and tenacity.

The body's lubrication and structure are governed by kapha. It is in charge of the immune system, body fluid management, and tissue growth and development. Kapha also affects resilience to stress and emotional stability. People who have a balanced Kapha have robust immunity, calmness, and stability in their bodies. They have the capacity to properly nurture both themselves and others. On the other hand, disorders including sadness, lethargy, congestion, and weight gain can result from an imbalance in the Kapha. Kapha types need to be intellectually active to prevent stagnation, eat light, warming meals, and exercise frequently to keep their bodies in balance.

Each person has a distinct constitution, or Prakriti, which is determined by the interaction of the three doshas. People who have a mix of two doshas, called dual-dosha types (e.g., Vata-Pitta, Pitta-Kapha, or Vata-Kapha), are prevalent even if one dosha may be predominant. Making dietary and lifestyle decisions that support health and well-being is made easier when one is aware of their dosha constitution. Furthermore, dietary patterns, environmental conditions, stress levels, and seasonal variations can all affect the doshas, causing imbalances that require the use of suitable therapies.

Ayurvedic practitioners advise individualized methods that consider each person's distinct constitution and present condition in order to balance the doshas. It's important to keep things warm and regular for Vata types. They gain from a regimen that consists of consistent meals, enough sleep, and calming and grounding activities. Vata's chilly and dry characteristics may be balanced with warm, prepared dishes high in healthful fats and spices like cinnamon and ginger. Techniques like light yoga, meditation, and oil massage (abhyanga) are also helpful.

Pitta types have to control their natural intensity and heat. For balance to be maintained, cooling behaviors are crucial in both diet and lifestyle. Pitta's fiery temperament may be subdued by cooling and hydrating foods like cucumbers, melons, and leafy greens. It's crucial to stay away from extreme temperatures, spicy meals, and stressful circumstances. Pitta may be managed by partaking in relaxing activities like swimming, going on nature walks, and practicing mindfulness. Herbs like fennel, coriander, and aloe vera can also be added for their cooling properties.

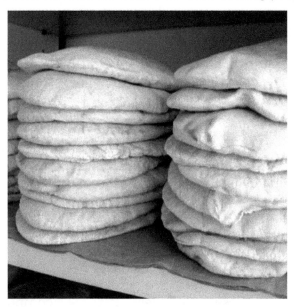

The priorities for kapha types should be increasing their metabolism and minimizing extra weight. Kapha's inherently heavy and damp nature may be countered by a diet rich in light, warm, and dry foods. Spices that improve digestion and metabolism include cumin, turmeric, and black pepper. For Kapha people, regular exercise is essential to avoiding stagnation and sustaining energy levels. Kapha's propensity for attachment and lethargy can be balanced by participating in novel and stimulating activities, dry brushing, and intense exercise.

Ayurvedic medicine uses a variety of therapies and treatments in addition to dietary and lifestyle guidelines to balance the doshas. Panchakarma is a rejuvenation and detoxification therapy that aims to remove toxins and bring the body and mind back into equilibrium. Herbal oil massages, thermal baths, and purifying methods like therapeutic vomiting (vamana) and nasal irrigation (nasya) are some of the treatments that are involved in this practice. Panchakarma is a systemic rejuvenation technique that is customized based on an individual's dosha constitution and existing imbalances.

Another essential component of Ayurvedic treatment is herbal medicine. Certain plants are utilized to treat different health issues and balance the doshas. For instance, Amalaki and neem are used to balance Pitta; ginger and turmeric are good for regulating Kapha, while ashwagandha and licorice root are frequently suggested for balancing Vata. These herbs can be taken in many different forms, including teas, powders, and capsules. To maximize their medicinalbenefits, these herbs are frequently combined in formulations.

External therapies like Shirodhara, which involves applying heated oil to the forehead to relax the nervous system and mind, and Basti, which involves using herbs to cleanse the colon and balance Vata, are also included in Ayurvedic treatments. These therapies offer a comprehensive approach to reestablishing balance and fostering well-being since they are carefully selected based on the individual's dosha constitution and particular health needs.

Ayurvedic principles affect not just an individual's health but also more general areas of life, including daily routines (dinacharya), seasonal rituals (ritucharya), and moral behavior (Advaita). Dinacharya offers advice on daily routines, such as getting up early, engaging in self-care rituals, and keeping a balanced schedule. Ritucharya offers instructions on how to adjust to seasonal variations, stressing the significance of modifying food and lifestyle to conform to the environment's natural cycles. Sadvritta is a comprehensive system of morality and social behavior that encourages harmony and balance in one's relationships with others and the environment.

In conclusion, knowledge of the qualities of the three doshas—Pitta, Kapha, and Vata—is essential to comprehend the fundamentals of Ayurvedic therapy. Vata, the element of lightness and mobility, regulates the body's ability to move and communicate. Heat-loving and intense, Pitta controls metamorphosis and metabolism. Kapha gives structure and lubrication; he is the embodiment of stability and wetness. The interaction of these doshas determines a person's constitution as well as their state of mind, body, and soul. People can attain maximum health and well-being by identifying and balancing their doshas through customized dietary, lifestyle, and treatment methods. The age-old knowledge of Ayurveda provides a thorough and all-encompassing foundation for comprehending the intricacies of human nature and encouraging balance and harmony in all facets of life.

How to identify your primary dosha

One of the cornerstones of Ayurvedic medicine, an age-old holistic health system that has its roots in India and dates back more than 5,000 years, is determining your predominant dosha. According to Ayurveda, each person is born with a distinct combination of the three doshas (Pitta, Kapha, and Vata), which dictate their mental, emotional, and physical traits. To attain and preserve balance, knowing your major dosha can help you make wise choices regarding your nutrition, way of life, and health regimen. This section examines the procedures and approaches for determining your primary dosha, such as self-evaluation, observing psychological and physical characteristics, and seeking expert advice.

First things first, it's important to comprehend the fundamental characteristics of the three doshas. Vata is represented by the components of air and space and is characterized by dryness, lightness, coolness, roughness, subtlety, and movement, among other attributes. Individuals with a strong Vata dosha usually have chilly extremities, dry, rough skin, and a fragile, thin physical structure. They may have erratic energy levels and frequently have unpredictable eating and sleeping schedules. Vata types are imaginative, quick-witted, and passionate in their thoughts, but they can also be prone to worry restlessness, and trouble focusing.

The fire and water parts of the pitta dosha give rise to attributes like heat, sharpness, intensity, and fluidity. Pitta dosha dominant people often have a medium frame, well-defined muscles, warm skin, and an inclination to perspire readily. They have a robust appetite, good digestion, and frequent episodes of hunger and thirst. Pitta types have sharp minds and are determined and well-organized, but they may also be easily agitated, impatient, and angry.

The characteristics of kapha dosha include weight, stability, smoothness, and wetness. It is connected to the elements of earth and water. Individuals with a prominent Kapha dosha are often strong and muscular, with smooth, oily skin and a composed steady manner. They frequently acquire weight and have slower metabolisms. Mentally, Kapha types are kind, understanding, and caring, yet they may also be clumsy, unyielding, and depressed.

One useful method for determining your primary dosha is self-assessment. This method entails analyzing your mental, emotional, and physical traits to ascertain which dosha dominates your constitution. You may use a variety of online tests and surveys to assist you in this self-evaluation process. Your body type, skin texture, hunger, digestion, energy levels, sleep habits, and emotional inclinations are all often questioned by these technologies. You can learn more about your primary dosha by being honest in your answers to these questions.

Another good way to figure out your major dosha is to observe your physical characteristics. Every dosha, as was previously noted, has unique physical traits. Vata types, for instance, typically have light, slender frames, noticeable veins and joints, and rough, dry skin. They could also exhibit unpredictable sleep habits and weak or irregular appetites. Generally speaking, Pitta types are medium-built, with moderately muscular bodies and warm, oily skin. They frequently have powerful appetites and digestive systems, and when these are out of balance, they may have rashes or acid reflux. Typically, kapha types are huge and robust, with thick hair and smooth, oily skin. Although they often have a constant hunger, they may digest food slowly, which can result in weight gain and lethargic behavior.

There are hints about your major dosha also found in your mental and emotional qualities. Vata people have a propensity for uneasiness and restlessness but are also frequently imaginative and quick-witted. They could have trouble focusing for long stretches of time and are frequently sidetracked. Although Pitta people are often goal-oriented, clever, and determined, they may also be easily agitated and angry. They are frequently born leaders with a clear sense of purpose. Although they have a propensity toward complacency and stubbornness, kapha people are often calm, patient, and caring. They might be sluggish to get going on new tasks, but once they do, they are trustworthy and consistent.

To have a more precise and thorough understanding of your major dosha, speaking with an Ayurvedic practitioner might be beneficial in addition to self-assessment and observation. Ayurvedic doctors are skilled in assessing a person's dosha constitution by using a variety of diagnostic methods, such as tongue analysis, pulse diagnosis, and in-depth inquiries regarding lifestyle, habits, and medical history. Ayurvedic practitioners use a historic technique called pulse diagnosis, or Nadi Pariksha, to determine the dosha balance by feeling the patient's radial pulse. Every dosha has its own unique pulse rhythm, and an adept practitioner may use the pulse's characteristics to determine imbalances.

Another diagnostic method employed by Ayurvedic doctors is tongue examination. The tongue's color, texture, coating, and any abnormalities can all reveal important details about the dosha's current condition. A tongue that is red and inflamed can point to a Pitta imbalance, whereas a tongue that is dry and cracked might point to a Vata imbalance. A thick layer of white coating on the tongue might indicate an imbalance of Kapha.

Asking insightful questions is another crucial step in the diagnosis procedure. Your daily schedule, eating habits, exercise regimen, sleep quality, and emotional inclinations will all be questioned by the practitioner. By asking these questions, the practitioner can better understand your lifestyle and how your dosha balance is affected. An Ayurvedic practitioner may provide a customized assessment of your major dosha and customized recommendations to improve your health and well-being by combining various diagnostic procedures.

When determining your major dosha, seasonal and environmental elements should be considered since they can also have an impact on your dosha balance. Seasons and environmental factors are linked to each dosha and can either exacerbate or alleviate its characteristics. The fall and early winter months, with their dry, chilly, and windy weather, are usually the worst for Vata dosha. People with mostly Vata dosha could feel more restless, anxious, and dry at this period. Vata has to be balanced; thus, it's critical to maintain warmth, hydration, and grounding through activities like eating warm, nutritious meals and doing peaceful things.

The hot and muggy summer months typically irritate the Pitta dosha. People with a prominent Pitta dosha may feel hotter, more irritable, and more inflammatory during this period. Pitta must be balanced by staying hydrated and cool, which may be achieved by doing soothing activities, avoiding extreme heat, and ingesting cooling foods and drinks.

The chilly, wet, and heavy weather of late winter and early spring tends to worsen Kapha dosha. People with mostly Kapha dosha may feel more congested and lethargic and may gain weight during this period. It is crucial to maintain warmth, movement, and stimulation—practices include eating light, warming meals, and exercising frequently—to balance Kapha.

Knowing how seasonal and environmental elements affect your dosha balance can help you make year-round, well-informed decisions regarding your nutrition and way of living. You may support your major dosha and keep your health and well-being at their best by modifying your routines and practices to suit the varying seasons.

The doshas are mostly balanced by food, and knowing which dosha is your predominant one can help you make dietary decisions that are compatible with your particular constitution. Certain food kinds are beneficial to each dosha and aid in preserving harmony and balance. Vata people should eat meals that are warm, wet, and grounded to balance out the dry and light characteristics of Vata. Warm soups, cooked grains, root vegetables, and healthy fats like olive oil and ghee are a few examples. Vata may also be balanced, and the digestive system is supported by spices like cumin, cinnamon, and ginger.

Foods that are cooling, moisturizing, and low in spice are beneficial to Pitta persons as they balance out the fiery and strong aspects of Pitta. Fresh produce, leafy greens, whole grains, and dairy products like milk and yogurt are a few examples. Spices and herbs like mint, fennel, and coriander can help calm and temper Pitta's fiery character. Additionally, excessive coffee, alcohol, and spicy meals that may worsen their dosha should be avoided by Pitta people.

Light, warm, and stimulating meals balance the heavy and moist features of the Kapha and are thus beneficial to those who are Kapha folks. Light grains like quinoa and barley, fresh produce, legumes, and seasonings like black pepper, ginger, and turmeric are a few examples. For Kapha people, it's critical to stay away from heavy, greasy, and sugary foods in order to keep their metabolisms healthy and avoid stagnation. Eating smaller meals or fasting frequently might also aid in balancing the Kapha.

A healthy lifestyle is important for balancing the doshas in addition to eating. Certain exercises and activities that complement each dosha's distinct composition are beneficial. Setting up routines is essential for Vata people to stay in equilibrium. This entails having regular mealtimes and sleep schedules as well as partaking in peaceful and centering pursuits like yoga, meditation, and leisurely strolls through the outdoors. Vata imbalances may be avoided by limiting travel, multitasking, and stimulating activities.

Activities that encourage emotional equilibrium, calming down, and relaxing are beneficial for Pitta people. This entails taking regular breaks, going outside, and indulging in peaceful pursuits like mindfulness meditation, tai chi, and swimming. Pitta people should also stay away from intense rivalry, overindulgence in labor, and exposure to heat and sunshine.

Activities that provide diversity, mobility, and excitement are beneficial to Kapha personalities. This entails exercising often, experimenting with different pastimes and pursuits, and including energizing routines like dancing, dry brushing, and aerobic workouts. Kapha equilibrium requires avoiding overeating, sleeping in excess, and leading sedentary lives.

Self-care routines that you include in your daily schedule can also help maintain dosha balance and general well-being. Warm oil is massaged over the body in a classic Ayurvedic technique called abhyanga, or self-oil massage, to nourish the skin, soothe the nervous system, and encourage circulation. You can use sesame oil for Vata, coconut oil for Pitta, and mustard or sunflower oil for Kapha, depending on your predominant dosha.

To sum up, determining your major dosha is a combination of self-evaluation, observing psychological and physical characteristics, and seeking expert advice. Knowing the traits of the Vata, Pitta, and Kapha doshas enables you to identify the dosha that predominates in your constitution and to make well-informed choices regarding your lifestyle, nutrition, and medical habits. By synchronizing your daily schedule, nutritional preferences, and self-care regimen with your distinct dosha constitution, you may attain and preserve equilibrium, promoting maximum health and wellness. The age-old knowledge of Ayurveda provides a thorough and individualized method for recognizing and fostering the intricacies of human nature, encouraging balance and vigor in all facets of life.

Imbalances and their effects on health

A multifaceted concept that encompasses physical, mental, and social well-being is health. Numerous health problems might arise when the delicate equilibrium within these dimensions is upset. A number of factors, including dietary inadequacies, hormone imbalances, mental health conditions, and lifestyle decisions, can cause imbalances. Having a thorough understanding of these imbalances and how they affect health is essential to developing plans to preserve general well-being.

Nutritional imbalances are among the most prevalent imbalances that have an impact on health. Numerous health issues can arise from either an excess or a deficiency in nutrients. For instance, diseases like rickets, scurvy, and anemia can result from a diet low in important elements like vitamins and minerals. One of the most common nutritional illnesses, iron deficiency anemia, is caused by inadequate intake or absorption of iron and manifests as weakness, exhaustion, and reduced cognitive function. Similarly, scurvy, which manifests as weariness, joint pain, and bleeding gums, can be brought on by a deficiency of vitamin C. Conversely, overconsumption of specific nutrients, such as sugars and fats, can lead to diabetes, obesity, and cardiovascular disorders. An ongoing imbalance in calories results in weight gain that raises the risk of heart disease, stroke, type 2 diabetes, and other chronic disorders. Thus, avoiding these health problems and enhancing general well-being needs eating a balanced diet.

Unbalances in hormones also have a big impact on health. These substances are messenger compounds that regulate many bodily functions, so changes in their amounts may have a big effect. For example, disorders like hypothyroidism and hyperthyroidism can result from an imbalance in thyroid hormones. The condition known as hypothyroidism, which is defined by inadequate thyroid hormone synthesis, can result in symptoms including sadness, tiredness, weight gain, and decreased cognitive performance. On the other hand, overproduction of thyroid hormone, or hyperthyroidism, can cause palpitations, anxiety, heat sensitivity, and weight loss. Diabetes is another frequent hormonal imbalance in which the body either cannot use the insulin it generates efficiently or does not make enough of it. This imbalance results in high blood sugar, which can lead to major problems, including neuropathy, retinopathy, and cardiovascular disease, if improperly handled. Menopause and polycystic ovarian syndrome (PCOS) are two examples of hormonal abnormalities linked to reproductive health that can have a significant impact on both physical and mental health. For instance, PCOS is linked to infertility, irregular menstrual periods, and a higher risk of metabolic problems. Thus, preserving health and avoiding long-term consequences need an awareness of and approach to hormone abnormalities.

Unbalances in mental health are another important factor that can have a big influence on general health. Mental health imbalances, including depression, anxiety, bipolar illness, and schizophrenia, impact millions of individuals globally. Depression can cause physical symptoms such as weariness, changes in appetite, and sleep difficulties. Depression is defined by persistent feelings of sorrow, despair, and loss of interest. Excessive concern and dread are the hallmarks of anxiety disorders, which can manifest physically as palpitations, perspiration, and digestive problems. Extreme mood fluctuations between mania and sadness are a feature of bipolar disease that can cause disruptions to everyday activities and, during manic episodes, dangerous behaviors. A severe mental illness called schizophrenia can lead to delusions, hallucinations, and problems with cognition. These mental health disorders have a greater impact on a person's relationships, productivity, and physical health, in addition to their quality of life. Long-term stress can exacerbate pre-existing medical conditions, weaken the immune system, and increase the risk of cardiovascular diseases. It is connected to mental health issues as well. Consequently, enhancing general health and well-being requires treating mental health imbalances through counseling, medication, and supporting treatments.

Significant contributions to health imbalances are also made by environmental variables and lifestyle decisions. For example, physical inactivity is a major contributing reason for obesity, heart conditions, and numerous forms of cancer. On the other hand, regular exercise helps you maintain a healthy weight, strengthens your heart, and improves your mental well-being. Unhealthy eating choices, such as consuming large quantities of processed foods, sweets, and unhealthy fats, can raise the risk of developing chronic illnesses and cause nutritional imbalances. It is commonly recognized that smoking and excessive alcohol use cause lung cancer, cardiovascular issues, and liver damage. Lack of sleep, which is frequently disregarded, can deteriorate immune system strength, lower cognitive function, and raise the risk of mental health issues. Environmental variables can also worsen health imbalances, including exposure to poisons, pollution, and stressful living situations. For example, there is a greater chance of respiratory disorders, heart issues, and some types of cancer if one lives in a polluted area. Thus, preventing health imbalances and enhancing general well-being requires leading a healthy lifestyle and limiting exposure to detrimental environmental variables.

Social determinants of health, such as socioeconomic position, education, work, and access to healthcare, can also lead to imbalances. People from poorer socioeconomic origins frequently have less access to secure housing, wholesome food, and high-quality healthcare. A higher prevalence of chronic illnesses, mental health issues, and generally worse health outcomes can result from these discrepancies. Since education affects income levels, work prospects, and health literacy, it is crucial to one's health. A greater percentage of education is associated with improved health outcomes because it provides people with the knowledge and resources they need to make wise health decisions. Workplace safety, job security, and stress levels associated with the job all have an influence on employees' physical and mental health. Employment and working circumstances also have an impact on health. Another important factor is access to healthcare, as prompt and reasonably priced medical attention is necessary for both controlling and avoiding health imbalances. Untreated diseases, delayed diagnosis, and increased rates of morbidity and death can all be caused by disparities in access to healthcare. In order to promote fairness in health outcomes and lessen health disparities, it is imperative that these social determinants of health be addressed.

Additionally, as specific genetic mutations and hereditary illnesses might predispose people to certain health difficulties, genetic factors can also contribute to imbalances in health. People who have a family history of certain malignancies, diabetes, or cardiovascular disorders, for instance, may be more likely to develop these illnesses. Genetic disorders, including sickle cell anemia, Huntington's disease, and cystic fibrosis, which can significantly impair health and quality of life, are directly caused by hereditary genetic abnormalities. Making educated health decisions and taking preventative action can be facilitated by providing genetic testing and counseling to assist individuals in understanding their genetic predispositions. Furthermore, improvements in personalized medicine—which adjusts medical care to a patient's unique genetic composition—have the potential to more successfully address health imbalances.

In summary, imbalances in a range of health-related domains, including as diet, hormones, mental health, lifestyle, social factors, and genetics, can significantly impact an individual's overall state of health. Hormonal imbalances can cause physiological disturbances and raise the risk of metabolic illnesses, while nutritional imbalances can result in excesses or deficiencies that fuel chronic diseases. Inequalities in mental and physical health have a substantial influence on both lifestyle decisions and environmental variables also play a role in creating health inequalities. Socially constructed factors of being healthy, such as socioeconomic status and access to healthcare, have a considerable impact on health outcomes. Furthermore, hereditary predisposition to certain health issues might be attributed to genetic variables, underscoring the significance of preventative and customized therapy. Promoting general health and well-being requires addressing these imbalances through all-encompassing healthcare, wholesome lifestyle choices, and supporting interventions. People may actively take measures to have a balanced and healthy existence by being aware of and regulating these imbalances.

CHAPTER II

The Ayurvedic Approach to Nutrition

Food as medicine

Food was viewed as both nourishment and a vital tool for preserving health and curing illnesses in ancient societies, which is where the idea of using food as medicine originated. The saying "Let substance be your medicine as well as your medicine be thy nourishment," attributed to Hippocrates, highlights the intimate connection between diet and well-being. Food may be highly helpful in enhancing overall health, increasing the body's defense, and preventing the chance of acquiring chronic illnesses when chosen correctly.

Food serves as medicine mostly through its ability to prevent chronic illnesses. A diet rich in produce, whole grains, fruits, lean meats, and healthy fats can help lower the risk of heart disease, diabetes, and numerous cancers. Vegetarian and fruit products are rich in antioxidants, minerals, and essential vitamins that protect against both inflammation and oxidative stress, which are primary variables that contribute to chronic disease. Berries, for example, include antioxidants called anthocyanins that have been demonstrated to lower inflammation and enhance cardiovascular health. Similarly, leafy greens high in vitamins A, C, and K, such as spinach and kale, support strong bones and a robust immune system. Similarly, leafy greens high in vitamins A, C, and K, such as spinach and kale, support strong bones and a robust immune system. Ancient grains such as quinoa-grown brown rice and millet are among the best sources of fiber, which helps lower cholesterol, regulate blood sugar, and support the functioning of the gut. Omega-3 fatty acids are very good for heart health and have anti-inflammatory qualities. They are mostly present in fatty fish, such as salmon and mackerel. When people regularly consume these nutrient-dense meals, their chance of acquiring chronic illnesses can be greatly decreased.

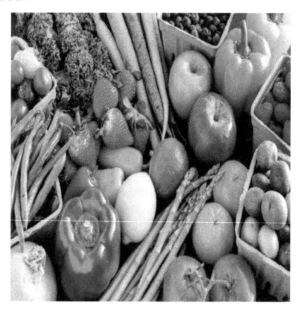

Food plays an equally important part in addressing pre-existing health issues. Making the right food choices is essential for diabetics to keep their blood glucose levels stable. Insulin sensitivity may be controlled, and blood sugar spikes can be avoided with a diet high in fiber, healthy fats, and complex carbs and low in processed sweets. Whole grains, legumes, and non-starchy vegetables are examples of low-glycemic diets that help maintain stable blood sugar levels because they release glucose into the bloodstream more gradually. Dietary measures to Stop a type of hyper or DASH diet places a strong emphasis on reducing salt intake while increasing intake of fresh produce, whole grains, vegetables, protein-rich foods, and reduced-fat dairy items. According to studies, those with hypertension who follow the DASH diet have much lower blood pressure, which lowers their risk of heart disease and stroke. In a similar vein, foods high in soluble fiber, such as oats, beans, and apples, can help lower LDL (bad) cholesterol levels in those with elevated cholesterol. Enhancing lipid profiles can also benefit from the inclusion of heart-healthy fats such as those found in almonds, avocados, and olive oil. These instances show how food may be an effective tool for controlling and enhancing medical problems.

Beyond the prevention and treatment of chronic illnesses, nutrition is essential for boosting immune system performance. A well-balanced diet rich in various nutrients supports the body's defenses to fight against viral and bacterial infections. Particular nutrients, such as the minerals selenium and zinc, vitamin C, and the hormone vitamin D, are very important for the function of the immune system. Fruits such as citrus, broccoli, red bell peppers, and berries are foods strong in vitamin C, which is widely recognized for boosting immunity. Fortified dairy products, fatty fish, and sunshine exposure are good sources of vitamin D, which is necessary for immunological modulation and has been associated with a lower incidence of respiratory infections. The immune system's operation and the healing of wounds depend on zinc. Foods including meat, fish, beans, and seeds may contain it. Good sources of the element selenium, an antioxidant that supports the defense function and helps protect cells from damage, include nuts, seeds, and shellfish. Probiotics, which are included in fermented foods like yogurt, kefir, sauerkraut, and kimchi, not only provide these nutrients but also support a healthy gut microbiota, which is essential for immune system function. Since many of the body's immune cells reside in the gut, keeping the gut's bacterial balance in check helps strengthen the body's defense. People can enhance their resistance to infections and fortify their immune systems by eating a varied and nutrient-rich diet.

Food has the therapeutic ability to improve mental health as well. Recent studies indicate that nutrition has a major impact on mental health, mood, and cognitive performance. An important factor in this relationship is the gut-brain axis, a bidirectional communication network that connects the two organ systems. Reducing inflammation, controlling the synthesis of neurotransmitters, and building stress resistance are just a few of the ways that a diet high in fiber, prebiotics, and probiotics can maintain a healthy gut microbiota and improve mental health. Fatty acids such as omega-3, which have been demonstrated to have anti-inflammatory properties and mitigate the hallmarks of anxiety and depression, are found in abundance in walnuts, fatty fish, and flaxseeds. Moreover, complex carbohydrates, such as those found in vegetables, legumes, and healthful grains, can help control the level of blood sugar and provide a steady source of energy, reducing irritability and mood fluctuations. For the health of the brain and regulation of mood, other vitamins and minerals are also necessary, such as minerals like magnesium, iron and B vitamins. B vitamins, which are required for the synthesis of neurotransmitters and energy, are found in entire grains, dark-colored vegetables, and lean meats. Magnesium calms the neurological system and can assist with the symptoms of anxiety and sadness. It can be found in nuts, seeds, and dark chocolate. Red meat, lentils, and fortified cereals are good sources of iron, which is necessary for the brain's oxygen delivery system and general cognitive function. People can improve their general quality of life and promote their mental health by providing these nutrients to their bodies.

Aside from its obvious health advantages, mindful eating—which involves giving your whole attention to the meal—can also enhance general well-being. Making thoughtful meal choices, appreciating food, and recognizing hunger and fullness cues are all encouraged by mindful eating. This strategy can promote a better relationship with food, lessen overeating, and enhance digestion. People may enjoy meals more and feel less stressed about their eating habits by taking the time to slow down and enjoy the sensory components of eating. A better understanding of the body's nutritional requirements is another benefit of mindful eating, which helps people make more balanced and healthier food choices. This all-encompassing method of eating promotes mental and emotional wellness in addition to physical health.

Furthermore, the therapeutic benefits of food have long been acknowledged by integrative and conventional medical approaches. For instance, meals are categorized in Ayurvedic medicine according to their energetic qualities and how they affect the body's doshas or basic energies. This antiquated method places a strong emphasis on the value of a balanced diet that is customized to each person's constitution and health requirements. In a similar vein, food is seen by Traditional Chinese Medicine (TCM) as a tool for promoting harmony among the body's organ systems and yin and yang energy balance. TCM practitioners frequently suggest particular foods and herbs to improve general well-being and treat health problems. These customs demonstrate the ingrained belief that food can heal and offer insightful information about the possible therapeutic benefits of dietary choices.

The push for using food as medicine in the current day also highlights the significance of environmental health and sustainability. Consuming organic, locally grown, and minimally processed food are examples of sustainable eating habits that are good for the environment as well as for human health. The use of pesticides, monocropping, and excessive water use in industrial agricultural methods have a negative influence on the environment and lead to soil erosion, water pollution, and biodiversity loss. People may lessen their ecological footprint and support agricultural methods that improve environmental health by selecting foods that have been produced responsibly. Furthermore, studies have demonstrated that plant-based diets, which prioritize eating enough fruits, vegetables, legumes, nuts, and seeds, have less of an adverse effect on the environment than diets heavy on animal products. Cutting back on meat consumption and increasing your intake of plant-based meals will help protect the environment, alleviate climate change, and improve animal welfare. The relationship between individual health and environmental sustainability highlights the wider effects of dietary practices and the cumulative effect of food choices on the environment.

In summary, the idea of food as medicine recognizes the significant influence that dietary decisions have on one's physical, mental, and environmental health and incorporates a holistic approach to health and well-being. A diet rich in nutrients can help manage and avoid chronic illnesses, strengthen the immune system, improve mental health, and advance general well-being. This method is further enhanced by the incorporation of traditional medical concepts and the mindful eating practice, which promotes a stronger bond with food and its restorative qualities. Furthermore, sustainable food practices emphasize the connection between environmental sustainability and human health, highlighting the significance of mindful food choices for the health of people and the environment. People may actively pursue optimal health and make a positive impact on a better, more sustainable world by adopting the concept of food as medicine.

Importance of digestion and Agni (digestive fire)

Food is broken down into nutrients during digestion, a basic process that keeps life alive. The body needs these nutrients for growth, energy production, and cellular repair. This notion is furthered by the Ayurvedic idea of Agni, or digestive fire, which emphasizes the vital role that effective digestion plays in preserving general health. Agni, as per Ayurveda, is a potent energy that regulates metabolism, transformation, and vitality in addition to being a physical process. Agni is said to be vital to health, and when it is out of balance, it can cause a variety of illnesses. This section examines the significance of Agni and digestion, emphasizing their contributions to mental and physical wellness as well as the avoidance of illness.

The most basic step in the digestive process is the chemical and physical dissolution of food into components that may be absorbed. When food is digested and coupled with saliva that includes enzymes like amylase, carbs are broken down in the mouth. After passing down the esophagus, the meal enters the stomach, where pepsin and hydrochloric acid, among other gastric secretions, further break down proteins. When the food reaches the small intestine, the enzymes from the pancreas and bile complete its breakdown, allowing the blood to take in the nutrients. After being absorbed by the large intestine, where water and minerals are taken up, the leftover indigestible food wastes are finally expelled.

Good digestion is essential for absorbing nutrients and maintaining general health. When digesting is at its peak, nutrients such as amino acids, vitamins, minerals, and lipids are effectively removed and distributed to cells across the body. Numerous biological processes, such as the manufacture of hormones, the creation of energy, the immune system, and tissue repair, depend on these nutrients. On the other hand, inadequate digestion can result in a lack of certain nutrients, which can cause weakness in the immune system, weariness, acne, and other health problems. For instance, low iron consumption can result in iron deficiency anemia, which can cause exhaustion and reduced cognitive function, while poor absorption of vitamin B12 can cause anemia and neurological issues.

In addition to the mechanical process, dietary habits, way of life, and stress all have an impact on digestion. Among the signs of a compromised digestive system brought on by an excessive intake of processed meals, sweets, and bad fats are bloating, constipation, and indigestion. On the other hand, a diet rich in veggies, whole grains, fruit, meat that is lean, and fiber and well-balanced ensures regular bowel movements and a functioning gastrointestinal system. Lifestyle elements like exercise, drinking enough of water, and getting enough sleep are also very important. Frequent activity promotes intestinal contractions, which facilitate the passage of food through the digestive tract; proper hydration maintains the proper functioning of the digestive system. The body, especially the digestive system, can heal and rebuild when it gets enough sleep. On the other hand, long-term stress can impede digestion by inducing the release of stress hormones like cortisol, which can impede or disturb digestive functions and result in disorders like irritable bowel syndrome (IBS).

The notion of Agni in Ayurvedic medicine broadens the definition of digestion to include not only the breakdown of food physically but also its conversion into energy and consciousness. Agni is seen as the fire of metabolism and digestion, turning food into nutrients that are accessible and getting rid of trash. Ayurveda states that there are three forms of Agni, each with a distinct function in the metabolic and digestive processes: Jatharagni (the fire in the stomach), Bhutagni (the elemental fire), and Dhatvagni (the tissue fire). The primary fire in the stomach and small intestine that controls the first stages of food digestion is called maharani. The five components of food—earth, water, fire, air, and ether—are processed by Bhutagni, while Dhatvagni converts nutrition into the seven body tissues (dhatus) of bone, marrow, plasma, muscle, fat, and reproductive tissue.

According to Ayurveda, a regulated Agni is necessary for good health and well-being. Digestion is successful, nutrients are correctly absorbed, and waste materials are effectively removed when Agni is robust and balanced. Ojas, or vitality, is the result of this equilibrium and is typified by robust immunity, mental clarity, and general well-being. On the other hand, weak Agni, also called Mandagni (weak fire), can result in poor digestion, the build-up of Ama (toxins), and a host of other health problems. Ama is regarded as a hazardous residue that develops from partially or incompletely digested food. Its build-up can clog body channels (srotas) and interfere with physiological processes, which can result in illness. Lethargy, indigestion, gas, bloating, and a coated tongue are signs of impeded Agni and Ama build-up.

Agni can be affected by a number of things, according to Ayurveda, including an unbalanced diet, erratic eating patterns, stress, and a sedentary lifestyle. Eating meals that are hard to digest, including processed, heavy, and greasy foods, can strain the digestive tract and deplete Agni. Agni can also be harmed by irregular eating schedules, overindulgence, and eating when not hungry. Physical, mental, or emotional stress can all have a big effect on Agni by detracting energy from digestion and inducing inflammation. Agni can be further weakened by a sedentary lifestyle, which lowers metabolic activity and damages circulation.

There are several food and lifestyle recommendations made by Ayurveda to maintain a balanced Agni. Eating warm, freshly cooked food that is readily digested is essential for Agni support. Spices that are believed to increase digestive fire and improve digestion include fennel, ginger, cumin, and coriander. Additionally, mindful eating—which includes digesting food completely, paying close attention to the experience of eating, and avoiding distractions like television or cell phones during meals—is another point of emphasis for Ayurveda. Important strategies for assisting Agni include eating in a quiet and comfortable setting, eating at regular times, and consuming sensible amounts of sizes. In addition, keeping a balanced Agni and general health requires frequent physical exercise, the use of stress-reduction methods like yoga and meditation, and enough sleep.

Ayurveda's connection between Agni and mental health is another important concept. Mental digestion, or the capacity to process ideas and emotions, is vital for mental health, much as physical digestion is for drawing nutrients from food. Agni promotes mental clarity, emotional stability, and an optimistic attitude toward life when it is in harmony. On the other hand, compromised Agni can result in mental dyspepsia, which manifests as disorientation, unease, despondency, and trouble focusing. According to Ayurveda, the mind and body are intertwined, and mental and physical well-being depend on having a balanced Agni.

Apart from food and lifestyle recommendations, Ayurveda provides a range of therapies to uplift Agni and enhance general well-being. The traditional Ayurvedic cleansing and rejuvenation treatment known as panchakarma seeks to eradicate Ama and bring Agni back into equilibrium. Massage, herbal steam therapy, and purging methods like Virechana (purgation) and Basti (medicated enema) are all part of this all-inclusive treatment. Panchakarma is usually performed under the supervision of a skilled Ayurvedic practitioner and is customized to each person's constitution and health requirements. To strengthen Agni and enhance digestion, herbal therapies like Triphala, a mixture of three fruits, and digestive formulations like Hingvastak Churna are also frequently utilized.

In summary, one cannot stress the significance of Agni, or digestive fire, and digestion for overall wellness. While inefficient digestion can result in a variety of health problems, efficient digestion is necessary for the body to produce energy, absorb nutrients, and maintain overall health. The Ayurvedic notion of Agni highlights the vital function that a healthy Agni plays in preserving health by expanding our knowledge of digestion to encompass the conversion of food into energy and consciousness. People can increase their physical and emotional well-being, minimize the build-up of pollutants, and promote effective digestion by implementing dietary and lifestyle behaviors that support Agni. Ayurveda's holistic approach to health, which incorporates diet, way of life, and medical procedures, sheds insight on the intimate connection between digestive system health and overall well-being. Although research on the complex link between digestion, nutrition, and health is still ongoing in modern science, the age-old knowledge of Ayurveda offers a timeless foundation for comprehending and maximizing this essential component of well-being.

Six tastes (sweet, sour, salty, bitter, pungent, astringent) and their effects

Awareness of nutrition and health requires an awareness of the six tastes, which are sweet, sour, salty, bitter, pungent, and astringent. This idea is derived from traditional Ayurvedic medicine. According to Ayurveda, these flavors are not just pleasing to the senses but also have an impact on one's mental, emotional, and physical well-being. The basic physical energies of the body, known as the doshas (Vata, Pitta, and Kapha), are influenced differently by each flavor and are linked to certain components. Maintaining health and avoiding disease requires a diet that balances these preferences. The six tastes, their origins, and their impacts on the body and mind are all examined in this section.

One of the most common tastes in human diets is sweetness, which is connected to the elements of earth and water. Naturally sweet foods include grains, fruits, dairy products, and certain vegetables, such as carrots and sweet potatoes. Sweet flavors are recognized for their ability to strengthen and nourish. It increases tissue construction, gives energy, and encourages growth and development. Because of its grounding and relaxing qualities, this flavor is good for lowering the Vata dosha, which is represented by components of air and space. Additionally, sweet meals have been shown to strengthen the immune system and improve skin tone. On the other hand, consuming too many sweets can cause imbalances, especially in the earthy and watery aspects of the Kapha dosha. Overindulgence in sugary meals can lead to obesity and diabetes, as well as weight gain and fatigue. Consequently, although sweetness is necessary for energy and fulfillment, it should only be used in moderation to prevent harmful consequences on one's health.

Foods like citrus fruits, fermented goods, and sour dairy items like yogurt include an earthy and fiery taste. Digestive enzyme release is increased by sour taste, which promotes hunger and digestion. Grounding and hydrating the body helps balance Vata dosha. However, excessive use of it might irritate Kapha and Pitta doshas. An excess of sour taste can upset the fire and water-related Pitta dosha, causing ailments like acid reflux, heartburn, and skin irritations. Similarly, for Kapha types, an overabundance of sour foods can cause edema, congestion, and water retention. The mind is likewise revitalized and refreshed by the sour taste; nevertheless, excessive ingestion may lead to agitation and frustration. In order to improve digestion and awaken the senses, the sour flavor should be incorporated into the diet; nevertheless, it must be balanced with other tastes to avoid dosha imbalances.

The most prevalent sources of the salty flavor are sea salt, rock salt, and naturally salty foods like seaweed. Salt is associated with the elements of fire and water. Salt is necessary to facilitate digestion, preserve electrolyte balance, and improve food flavor. It is helpful for calming the Vata dosha because of its warming and moisturizing properties. Salt increases hunger and facilitates nutrition absorption. On the other hand, consuming too much salt can exacerbate the Pitta and Kapha doshas, which can result in elevated inflammation, hypertension, and water retention. Consuming excessive amounts of salt can also aggravate renal problems and cardiovascular illnesses. Ayurveda believes that the taste of salt increases bravery and mental clarity; nevertheless, too much salt can lead to excessive thirst and agitation. Because of this, even while salt is essential for many body processes, it should only be taken sparingly to prevent negative health effects.

Foods like bitter melon, leafy greens, and some herbs and spices like fenugreek and turmeric include a bitter flavor, which is made up of ether and air constituents. Bitter flavors are recognized for their ability to purify and cleanse. It eases fever, promotes digestion, and aids in the body's removal of toxins. Foods that are bitter have cooling and drying properties that help lower the doshas of Pitta and Kapha. They encourage clarity and lightness, which can help counteract the heavy and congested qualities of Kapha. On the other hand, a diet high in bitter foods can exacerbate Vata dosha and cause symptoms like anxiety, dryness, and upset stomach. Additionally, helpful in lowering cravings for salty and sweet meals, the bitter flavor aids in weight control. Bitter foods have the potential to improve mental clarity and self-awareness, but they should be consumed in moderation to prevent negative thoughts and overstimulating the mind. Bitter foods are good for you in many ways, but to keep you healthy overall, you need to balance them with other flavors in your diet.

The fiery and spicy characteristics of the pungent flavor are linked to the components of air and fire. Pungent foods include specific vegetables like onions and garlic as well as spices like chili peppers, ginger, and black pepper. The strong flavor enhances circulation, releases congestion, and speeds up digestion. Because of its warming properties, it helps to balance the Kapha dosha in the body. Spicy meals are well-known for their capacity to speed up metabolism and eliminate pollutants. On the other hand, overindulgence can exacerbate Pitta and Vata doshas, resulting in symptoms like acidity, heartburn, and irritation. The strong flavor also stimulates the intellect, making one more focused and aware. However, eating too much spicy food might overstimulate, which can result in agitation and violence. Therefore, in order to avoid imbalances and maintain mental and physical equilibrium, it should only be used in moderation—even if the strong flavor is necessary for healthy digestion and metabolic processes.

Legumes, green apples, cranberries, and other vegetables, like broccoli and cauliflower, have an astringent flavor that is made up of earth and air ingredients. It is well-recognized that an astringent flavor may be cold and dry. It aids in absorbing more moisture, lowering inflammation, and accelerating recovery. This flavor gives a sensation of solidity and lightness, which is good for balancing the doshas of Pitta and Kapha. Eating meals high in tanning agents is another way to tighten tissues and enhance skin health. On the other hand, a diet high in astringent foods can exacerbate Vata dosha, causing anxiety, constipation, and dryness. An astringent flavor can improve mental focus and self-control, but if it isn't counterbalanced by other tastes, it can also cause emotions of rigidity and loneliness. To preserve general health and well-being, astringent meals should be taken in harmony with other tastes. Astringent foods can offer health advantages, including cleansing and tissue healing.

Ayurvedic teachings state that preserving health requires balancing the six flavors in the diet. A diverse range of tastes is consumed to ensure that all nutritional demands are satisfied and to promote equilibrium among the doshas. Each flavor has distinct qualities and effects on the body and mind. A meal that balances the flavors of sweet, sour, salty, bitter, pungent, and astringent ingredients, for example, can improve metabolic processes, improve digestion, and reduce food cravings. This well-rounded eating strategy offers complete sustenance for the body and mind in addition to pleasing the palate.

Seasonal eating also heavily relies on the six flavors. Ayurveda holds that the body's requirements vary with the seasons and that eating a diet that suits one's tastes may help one stay in balance and be healthy. For instance, to counteract the heat and avoid Pitta imbalances in the sweltering summer, cooling flavors like sweet, bitter, and astringent are advised. On the other hand, to aid in digestion and maintain Vata balance during the chilly winter months, warming flavors like sweet, salty, and aromatic are prioritized. People can improve their general well-being and increase their resistance to environmental stresses by coordinating their diet with seasonal variations.

In conclusion, a comprehension of nutrition and health from an Ayurvedic viewpoint requires an awareness of the six tastes: sweet, sour, salty, bitter, pungent, and astringent. Maintaining health and avoiding disease requires striking a balance between the flavors in the diet since each has distinct advantages and consequences on the body and mind. Astringent tastes absorb excess moisture and aid in healing, sour tastes stimulate digestion, salty tastes preserve electrolyte balance, and bitter tastes detoxify and cleanse. Sweet tastes nourish and strengthen. People can attain a balanced and harmonious state of health by responding to seasonal fluctuations and introducing a range of flavors into their diet. Gaining a better understanding and appreciation of the six tastes may help one appreciate food as a means of sustenance, healing, and general well-being.

Eating according to your dosha

Ayurvedic medicine is based on the core premise of individualizing food and lifestyle choices for maximum health and well-being. Eating in accordance with one's dosha is one way to do this. The traditional Indian healthcare system, referred to as Ayurveda, divides the doshas into three primary categories: Pitta, Kapha, and Vata. The five elements—earth, water, fire, air, and ether—represent distinct combinations in each dosha, which is linked to certain mental, emotional, and physical traits. You may make dietary decisions that support harmony and balance in your body and mind by being aware of your dominant dosha. This section examines the traits of each dosha and offers thorough advice on how to eat for good health based on your dosha.

Lightness, dryness, coolness, and movement are characteristics of the vata dosha, which is made up of air and ether. People who have a strong Vata dosha are frequently thin, have dry skin, and have fickle appetites. They are usually quick-witted, gregarious, and creative, but they can also be prone to restlessness, anxiety, and digestive problems like constipation and bloating. Eating warm, moist, nutritious, and grounding meals is essential for balancing Vata. Meals that are warm and prepared work best for Vata types since they balance out the dry and frigid characteristics of Vata. Warming spices like ginger, cumin, and cinnamon are especially good in soups, stews, and porridge. Avocados, ghee, and olive oil are examples of healthy fats that give moisture and nutrients, which help to relieve dryness. People with a vata constitution should abstain from cold, raw meals and drinks since they might exacerbate their already dry and frigid constitution. Maintaining a regular schedule and eating habits is also critical to balancing the innate vata fluctuation.

Heat, intensity, and sharpness are characteristics of the Pitta dosha, which is made up of fire and water. People with pitta traits frequently have a medium body type, a warm body temperature, and a voracious appetite. Although they are often driven, ambitious, and passionate, they can also be easily agitated and prone to inflammatory diseases like rashes and acid reflux. It is crucial to eat cooling, soothing, and tranquil foods to regulate Pitta. Fresh foods, especially ones high in moisture like cucumbers also melons, and leafy greens, can effectively cool down Pitta's heat. If dairy items like milk, yogurt, and ghee are eaten in moderation and aren't overly heavy or greasy, they can also help calm Pitta's fiery character. Pittas should choose flavors that are sweet, bitter, and astringent; they should stay away from meals that are too spicy, salty, or sour, as they will intensify their inner fire. Pitta balance also requires frequent mealtimes and abstaining from excessive stimulants like alcohol and coffee.

Heaviness, wetness, and stability are characteristics of the kapha dosha, which is made up of earth and water. People who are kapha tend to be larger in stature, have smooth skin, and have slower metabolisms. Although they can also be prone to tiredness, weight gain, and congestion, they are usually calm, patient, and caring. Eating light, dry, and stimulating meals is essential for balancing Kapha. Detoxification and lightening of the Kapha are aided by fresh, raw fruits and vegetables, especially those that are pungent, bitter, and astringent.

Ideal foods include leafy greens, berries, apples, and cruciferous vegetables like cauliflower and broccoli. In order to combat Kapha's lethargy, spices like ginger, black pepper, and turmeric can aid in boosting metabolism and digestion. Foods that are heavy, greasy, and sugary should be avoided by Kapha people since these foods might exacerbate their propensity for weight gain and congestion. Maintaining physical exercise and eating light, frequent, varied meals are also essential for preserving the Kapha equilibrium.

Apart from these broad dietary recommendations, Ayurveda also stresses the significance of mindful eating and matching food choices to the seasons. The dosha balance can be affected by the seasons; therefore, modifying your diet might help keep things in balance. For instance, Pitta dosha is inherently heightened during the hot summer months; to counterbalance this, consume cooling foods like salads, fresh fruits, and coconut water. On the other hand, Vata dosha tends to grow irritated in the chilly winter months. Warming, nutritious meals like soups, stews, and root vegetables can help keep the dosha in balance. Since springtime is linked to a rise in Kapha, lighter, detoxifying foods like legumes, greens, and sprouts can help lessen the heaviness of Kapha.

Eating to suit your dosha also requires mindful eating or giving your entire focus to the meal experience. This means sitting down to eat in a quiet and composed manner, chewing your food well, and enjoying the tastes and textures of your food. Eating mindfully facilitates a positive relationship with food, better digestion, and increased nutritional absorption. Additionally, it encourages you to focus on your body's feelings of fullness and hunger, which may assist you in choosing healthier foods and avoiding overindulging.

Additionally, Ayurveda acknowledges the significance of Agni, or digestion, in preserving general health. Food digestion, nutritional absorption, and waste removal are all accomplished by agna, also known as digestive fire. The buildup of poisons (Ama) and other health problems can result from an imbalanced Agni, which is necessary for optimum health. Every dosha affects Agni differently. Vata's irregularities can generate differing degrees of acidity in the body; Pitta's intensity can induce hyperacidity, and Kapha's heaviness can result in slow digestion. Eating in accordance with your dosha provides the right kinds of food and eating habits for your constitution, which supports balanced Agni.

Ayurveda considers not just the physical elements of eating but also the emotional and mental emotions that are associated with certain foods. Anxiety, stress, and bad feelings can upset the dosha equilibrium and hinder digestion. Enhancing digestion and promoting general well-being may be achieved via cooking and eating with mindfulness, gratitude, and good purpose. Eating may become a nutritious and restorative experience if you take a minute to breathe deeply, show thanks for the meal, and develop a good mentality.

The significance of food quality and preparation techniques is also emphasized by Ayurveda. Because they have more prana, or life force energy, meals that are fresh, organic, and locally produced are recommended. There is also an emphasis on using appropriate food preparation techniques, such as cooking with herbs and spices that improve digestion and nutritional absorption. For instance, incorporating fennel, ginger, and cumin into meals can help with digestion and minimize bloating and gas. Additionally, since processed and refined meals can be difficult to digest and lack essential nutrients, Ayurveda advises against consuming them.

Knowing what foods go together is a key component of eating to suit your dosha. While certain meal pairings might improve nutritional absorption and digestion, others can worsen digestion and produce toxins. For instance, Ayurveda discourages eating dairy products together with sour or citrus fruits as this might cause the dairy to curdle in the stomach and cause Ama. In a similar vein, eating fruit with meals is not advised since it breaks down fast and can ferment when combined with slower-digesting items. Toxin production may be avoided, and digestive equilibrium can be preserved by being aware of and adhering to the right dietary combinations.

Acknowledging and treating dietary allergies and sensitivities is another aspect of eating in accordance with your dosha. Certain sensitivities may be more common in each dosha. Vata people, for instance, may be sensitive to cold and raw meals; Pitta people, on the other hand, may be sensitive to spicy and acidic foods; and Kapha people to dairy and heavy foods. Maintaining balance and avoiding health problems need knowing which meals make you uncomfortable or produce negative reactions. In addition, Ayurveda provides a range of therapies and prescriptions, including customized meal plans, herbal formulations, and cleansing protocols, to manage food sensitivities and enhance digestive health.

To sum up, eating according to your dosha is a thorough approach to nourishment that considers the unique intellectual, physical, and emotional characteristics of each individual. You may enhance your overall health and well-being by being aware of your dominant dosha and choosing foods that balance it. Meals that are warm, moist, and grounding are beneficial to Vata doers; meals that are cooling, soothing, and relaxing are beneficial to Pitta doers; and foods that are light, dry, and stimulating are necessary for Kapha doers. Crucial components of this strategy include mindful eating, managing dietary sensitivities, adjusting for the season, and creating appropriate meal pairings. You may improve your general health and vigor and establish a harmonious connection with food by adhering to the principles of eating in accordance with your dosha.

Seasonal eating and its benefits

Seasonal dining is a long-standing custom that highlights the use of locally sourced and in-season foods. This nutritional strategy not only supports health, sustainability, and a wide variety of culinary options, but it also fits nicely with natural agricultural cycles. Seasonal eating has several advantages, including improved nutrition, fewer environmental effects, financial support for nearby farmers, and a stronger sense of community and connection to the natural world. This section examines the idea of seasonal eating and all of its advantages.

The concept of seasonal eating is based on the knowledge that different seasons yield different kinds of produce, each with special nutritional qualities catered to the body's needs at particular points in the year. For example, nature supplies an abundance of fruits and vegetables like melons, cucumbers, and leafy greens throughout the summer, when the temperature is hot and the body needs cooling and hydration. These meals help keep you hydrated because they are high in water content, and they also have cooling qualities that assist control body temperature. Conversely, root vegetables like sweet potatoes, carrots, and parsnips become more common in the winter when the body needs warmth and nourishment. These veggies are full of nutrients and calories, giving you the energy and calories, you need to stay warm.

The higher nutritious content of produce that is in season is one of the main advantages of eating seasonally. When fruits and vegetables are picked when they are at their ripest, they contain more antioxidants, vitamins, and minerals than when they are produced out of season. This is due to the fact that seasonal fruit is usually collected early and allowed to ripen naturally instead of being artificially ripened. For example, summer-picked tomatoes are often higher in nutrients and flavor than winter-picked ones. Research has indicated that foods that are in season may have higher concentrations of specific nutrients. For instance, spinach collected in the winter has more vitamin C than spinach collected in the summer. Therefore, eating seasonal produce guarantees that people get the most nutrients from their food.

Seasonal eating provides major environmental benefits in addition to nutritional ones. Eating locally farmed and in-season food decreases the environmental impact associated with food delivery and storage. Produce that is harvested outside of the season frequently has to be transported, refrigerated, and packaged in large quantities, all of which increase greenhouse gas emissions and damage the environment. People may reduce these effects and encourage more sustainable agriculture methods by selecting seasonal, locally sourced foods. Seasonal eating also promotes agricultural diversification. Rather than depending solely on a small number of in-demand goods, farmers are more likely to raise a diversity of crops all year round. This variety fosters a more robust and sustainable food system, lowers pest and disease cycles, and preserves the quality of the soil.

Seasonal eating also has significant financial advantages. Customers may help local farmers and the local economy by buying seasonal products. Farmers can boost their profits by selling directly to customers, cutting out middlemen. Small and family-run farms, which are frequently more community- and environmentally-focused than huge industrial farms, are supported financially by this financial assistance. Furthermore, since seasonal food doesn't need to be transported or stored, it is frequently less expensive than alternatives grown outside of the season. Customers may support their local communities financially while consuming fresher, more reasonably priced food.

Eating in season also promotes a closer relationship with the natural world and the earth's cycles. People who adjust their meals in accordance with the seasons have a greater awareness of the cycles of the natural world. Their appreciation of food and their level of awareness can both be improved by this relationship. As people modify their diets to reflect what is available throughout different seasons of the year, seasonal eating encourages people to try a greater range of foods and flavors. In addition to improving the dining experience, this range of cuisines encourages a more diversified and well-balanced diet. For instance, individuals may have fresh strawberries and asparagus in the spring and apples and pumpkins in the fall. This yearly rotation guarantees a wide range of nutrients and keeps the diet from becoming monotonous.

Additionally, eating in accordance with the seasons might improve mental and emotional health. Eating meals that are in line with the season and fresh, vivid flavors can improve energy and happiness. For example, the vibrant, juicy summer fruits may be energizing and refreshing, while the substantial, warming winter veggies can offer warmth and sustenance. Finding and cooking seasonal foods may also be a rewarding and pleasurable activity that strengthens one's bond with the land and the neighborhood.

In terms of cooking, seasonal eating encourages innovation and trial in the kitchen. Home cooks and chefs can experiment with new recipes and cooking methods based on the seasonal ingredients available. This technique promotes better eating habits in addition to improving the gastronomic experience. Meals made using seasonal vegetables are typically more healthful and nutrient-dense since they require less processing and additives. A delightful and simple summer salad featuring fresh tomatoes, cucumbers, and basil showcases the flavors of the season.

Around the world, cultural customs and behaviors are closely linked to seasonal eating. Many civilizations have distinct cuisines and delicacies that are connected to particular festivals or seasons. The seasonality of foodstuffs and the dietary requirements of the populace at that time are frequently reflected in these culinary customs. Mangoes in the summer and root vegetables in the winter are two examples of foods that are customarily consumed during festivals in India that correspond with the agricultural calendar. In nations around the Mediterranean, cuisine is seasonal, with lighter, fresher options during the warmer months and heartier, warming dishes during the cooler ones. Accepting seasonal eating enables people to understand the knowledge and wisdom ingrained in traditional diets and to establish a connection with these cultural traditions.

The promotion of food security and resilience is a noteworthy advantage of seasonal eating. An agricultural system that is both varied and locally oriented can withstand shocks like severe weather, unstable economies, and disruptions in the supply chain. Communities may strengthen and adapt their food system by consuming a range of seasonal foods and supporting local farmers. In light of climate change and other global issues that jeopardize food supply and availability, this resilience is especially crucial. Eating in season promotes sustainable agricultural methods that preserve the environment and guarantee the long-term viability of food production.

Seasonal eating is an opportunity to re-establish a connection with nature, boost local economies, and provide physical and mental nourishment in an increasingly convenience-driven society where sustainability and health are often neglected. It opposes the industrial food system's focus on consistency and year-round availability of all goods in favor of a more natural and well-rounded approach to eating. People may help create a healthier world and better version of themselves by choosing what and when to eat.

Putting seasonal eating patterns into practice may be simple and pleasurable. Begin by going to the farmers' markets in your area. These are great places to find seasonal, fresh produce. You may have a better knowledge and enjoyment of seasonal eating by talking to farmers and finding out when different crops are available. Planning meals around seasonal foods can be a creative and enjoyable experience, giving you the chance to try out new dishes and flavors. The advantages of eating seasonally may be extended throughout the year by preserving seasonal produce using techniques like canning, freezing, and fermenting. This way, there will always be a supply of wholesome foods available, even when they are not in season.

In summary, seasonal eating is a comprehensive and advantageous nutritional strategy that supports local businesses, encourages environmental sustainability, and corresponds with natural cycles. People may get more nutritional advantages, lessen their carbon footprint, and develop stronger ties to the environment and their community by eating crops that are in season. Eating in accordance with the seasons promotes culinary innovation and diversity, improves mental and emotional health, and increases resilience and food security. Adopting this technique provides a method to live a more happy, sustainable and health-conscious lifestyle. Seasonal eating offers timeless and invaluable guidance to nourishment for both the world and ourselves as we negotiate the intricacies of the contemporary food system.

CHAPTER III

Ayurvedic Kitchen Essentials

Common Ayurvedic spices and their healing properties

The traditional Indian medical discipline known as Ayurveda has long placed a strong emphasis on the role that nutrition and food play in preserving health and averting illness. The use of spices, which have several medicinal properties in addition to improving food flavor, is essential to this strategy. For millennia, common Ayurvedic spices like turmeric, ginger, cumin, coriander, fennel, black pepper, and cardamom have been used to support general well-being, improve immunity, and aid with digestion. This section examines these spices' therapeutic qualities as well as their applications in Ayurvedic medicine.

In Ayurveda, turmeric, or "haldi" as it is known in Hindi, is highly valued. Its primary ingredient, curcumin, is widely recognized for having potent anti-inflammatory and antioxidant qualities. Numerous illnesses, including arthritis, digestive issues, skin ailments, and respiratory infections, can be treated with turmeric. Turmeric is a multipurpose spice that may be used to support general health since it is thought to balance the three doshas of Pitta, Kapha, and Vata in Ayurvedic medicine. It improves skin tone, helps heal wounds, and promotes liver function. There are several ways to eat turmeric, including as tea, in meals, or as golden milk, an old Ayurvedic concoction of milk and spices.

"Adrak," or ginger, is another essential component of Ayurvedic therapy. This strong, warming spice is especially good for respiratory and digestive issues.

Ginger is useful in relieving bloating, nausea, and indigestion because it helps to promote Agni, the digestive fire. Its expectorant and anti-inflammatory qualities are also used to treat colds, coughs, and sore throats. Ginger helps relieve the pain and stiffness brought on by arthritis and muscular pains by improving circulation and lowering inflammation. In Ayurveda, ginger is frequently added to food to improve flavor and digestion. It can be ingested fresh, dried, or as a tea.

"Jeera," or cumin, is a widely prized spice for its digestive properties. Although its warming properties might occasionally worsen Pitta, it is especially useful in balancing the doshas of Vata and Kapha. Cumin stimulates digestive enzymes, which improves digestion and nutritional absorption. It is frequently used to ease bloating, gas, and pain in the abdomen. Additionally, cumin possesses antibacterial qualities that make it beneficial for immune system support and infection treatment. Cumin seeds are frequently dry-roasted in Ayurveda to intensify their flavor and strength before being used in a variety of recipes or blended into a calming tea for the digestive system.

The cooling spice coriander, also known as "dhaniya," is very helpful for regulating Pitta dosha. It works effectively to treat skin diseases, urinary tract infections, and digestive disorders, including indigestion and heartburn, because of its calming and purifying qualities. Ayurvedic cookery and medicine both employ coriander seeds and leaves. Fresh leaves may be added to foods for a burst of flavor and cooling impact, or the seeds can be cooked to produce a pleasant tea that helps with digestion and decreases inflammation. Additionally, well-known for its capacity to maintain healthy liver function and control blood sugar levels is coriander.

"Saunf," or fennel, is another cooling spice that is well-known for helping with digestion. It is very helpful in lowering Pitta and Vata doshas. Chewing fennel seeds after eating helps improve digestion by lowering gas, indigestion, and bloating while also freshening breath. Fennel tea is a well-liked Ayurvedic treatment for upset stomachs and helps nursing moms breastfeed. Fennel also contains diuretic qualities that aid in toxin removal and decrease water retention. Due to its mild, dulcet taste, it is a diverse pepper that performs well in savory as well as sweet recipes.

In Ayurveda, black pepper, or "kali mirch," is referred to as the "king of spices." Its capacity to improve metabolism and digestion makes it valuable. Black pepper is useful in treating indigestion, gas, and constipation because it increases the release of digestive enzymes. Its warming qualities balance the doshas of Kapha and Vata, but if taken in excess, they might worsen Pitta. Black pepper is frequently used in Ayurvedic formulations because it increases the bioavailability of other minerals and herbs. It is used to treat respiratory ailments, including colds and coughs, because of its antibacterial and anti-inflammatory qualities. In addition to being used in cooking, black pepper may be used in herbal teas and mixtures.

Ayurveda places great value on cardamom, also known as "elaichi," a sweet and fragrant spice with digestive and purifying qualities. It works particularly well to balance the doshas of Vata and Kapha. Cardamom eases nausea and vomiting, decreases gas, and promotes digestion. Because of its carminative qualities, it can help relieve bloating and pain in the abdomen. Cardamom is frequently used as a component in cough and cold medicines because of its reputation for clearing the lungs and enhancing respiratory health. Cardamom also has a relaxing impact on the mind, which is why it's frequently used to ease anxiety and enhance mental clarity. It may be steeped into a calming tea or incorporated into savory or sweet meals.

To maximize the medicinal benefits of these individual spices, Ayurvedic practitioners frequently utilize spice mixes like Trikatu and Chyawanprash. Trikatu is a mixture of dried ginger, long pepper (pippali), and black pepper that is believed to improve metabolism, promote digestion, and remove lung congestion. It works very well to balance the doshas of Vata and Kapha. The main component of chyawanprash, a classic Ayurvedic tonic, is amla (Indian gooseberry), which is combined with a number of other herbs and spices, such as cardamom, ginger, turmeric, and black pepper. This tonic helps the body regenerate, strengthen immunity, and improve digestion.

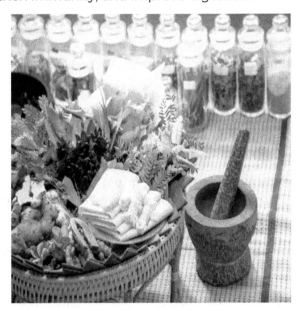

The application of spices in daily living is consistent with the holistic aspect of Ayurvedic therapy. In addition to being added to food, spices are also utilized in oils, pastes, and teas for medicinal purposes. Turmeric paste, for instance, is frequently applied externally to heal wounds and skin disorders, while ginger oil is used in massages to ease sore muscles and promote circulation.

Because of their adaptability, Ayurvedic spices may be employed in a multitude of ways to address a range of health issues.

Many of the ancient applications of Ayurvedic spices have been proven by contemporary scientific study, adding to their advantages. A compound that, the main component of turmeric, has been shown via research to have potent soothing and antibacterial properties that could potentially cure long-term illnesses including inflammation, arthritis, diabetes, and cardiovascular diseases. In a similar vein, ginger's digestive advantages and capacity to lessen nausea and vomiting—particularly in pregnancy and chemotherapy-induced nausea—have been the subject of much research. Spices like black pepper, cumin, and coriander have also been shown to possess antibacterial qualities, suggesting that they may be used to treat infections and boost immunity.

A simple and useful way to enhance your general health and well-being is to incorporate Ayurvedic spices into your diet. These easily accessible spices provide taste and nutrition to a variety of dishes. If you are new to Ayurvedic cuisine, you may get acquainted with the tastes and advantages of these spices by beginning with easy dishes that call for them. You may experiment with various preparations and combinations over time to find what suits your needs and tastes the best.

To sum up, typical Ayurvedic spices like cardamom, ginger, turmeric, cumin, coriander, fennel, and black pepper provide a plethora of therapeutic benefits that promote general health and well-being. These spices have been utilized for millennia in Ayurvedic medicine for treating a variety of disorders, such as inflammation, boosted immunity, and better digestion. Many of these historic usages are supported by modern scientific study, which emphasizes the natural medicines' potential for therapeutic use. You may take advantage of Ayurvedic spices' potent advantages and improve your general health by including them in your diet and way of life. These spices offer a flexible and all-encompassing approach to health and healing, whether they are employed in food preparation, drinks, or topical applications.

Staple ingredients in an Ayurvedic kitchen

Diet and nutrition play a major role in maintaining health and preventing disease in Ayurveda, the age-old Indian holistic medical system. An Ayurvedic kitchen is a veritable gold mine of basic foods that are selected for their therapeutic qualities as well as for nutritional worth. These components help maintain the equilibrium of the three doshas in the body—Pitta, Kapha, and Vata—which enhances general health and well-being. This section examines and highlights the relevance of the key components found in an Ayurvedic kitchen, such as grains, legumes, oils, spices, fruits, vegetables, dairy products, and herbs.

The foundation of an Ayurvedic diet, grains provide you with energy and nourishment. According to Ayurveda, rice, wheat, barley, and millet are some of the most sacred grains. Basmati rice, in particular, is thought to be extremely sattvic, which means it fosters mental clarity and purity. Since it is simple to digest, all doshas—Vata and Pitta in particular—can benefit from it. Whole wheat flour or split wheat is a grounding and nutritious grain that balances Pitta and Vata, but if taken in excess, it can irritate Kapha. Due to its light and dry nature, barley is good for the Pitta and Kapha doshas and is well-known for its diuretic characteristics. Gluten-free and light, millet is a cooling grain that balances Pitta and Kapha.

Another mainstay in Ayurvedic cooking, legumes are a great source of fiber and protein. Particularly well-liked are chickpeas, lentils, and mung beans. Because they may balance all three doshas, mung beans are regarded as tri-doshic. Since they are simple to digest and cleanse, cleansing diets frequently include them. All types of lentils—red, green, and yellow—are filling and adaptable, but improper preparation can make Vata rise. Although they might be heavy for Vata, chickpeas are nutritious and strong and good for balancing Pitta and Kapha. Legumes are frequently soaked and cooked with digestive spices such asafoetida, cumin, and coriander to improve digestion and lessen any possible aggravation of Vata.

Because of its medicinal qualities as well as its use as a cooking medium, oils are essential to Ayurvedic cookery. In Ayurveda, ghee, or clarified butter, is regarded as one of the most sattvic and therapeutic foods. All doshas can benefit from it, and it's well-recognized for boosting general vigor, enhancing nutrient absorption, and improving digestion. Although it might be too hot for Pitta doshas, sesame oil is warming and grounding, making it perfect for Vata and Kapha doshas. Because of its heavy nature, coconut oil should be used sparingly for Vata and Kapha. Its cooling and relaxing qualities make it ideal for Pitta balance. Another popular oil that is good for promoting digestion and regulating Kapha is mustard oil.

The main ingredient in Ayurvedic cookery, spices offer several health advantages in addition to flavor. Among the most utilized spices are cardamom, ginger, cumin, coriander, fennel, black pepper, and turmeric. Due to its well-known anti-inflammatory and antioxidant characteristics, turmeric supports immunity and general health. Ginger helps with respiratory problems, digestion, and inflammation reduction. Cumin aids in better digestion and intake of nutrients by optimizing the activity of enzymes that help with digestion. Cooling and cleansing, coriander is good for Pitta and urinary tract health. Fennel has a relaxing impact on the mind and aids with digestion and bloating reduction. In addition to improving the bioavailability of other nutrients, black pepper facilitates digestion. In addition to being calming, cardamom improves digestion, clears the air, and calms the mind.

Fruits and vegetables make up the majority of an Ayurvedic diet since they are high in nutritional content, minerals, and radicals. Produce grown locally and in season is best for optimum freshness and nutritional value. Commonly utilized foods include apples, pears, berries, melons, leafy greens, carrots, squash, and beets. Pears and apples are astringent and cooling, good for Pitta and Kapha. Due to their antioxidant content, berries are especially beneficial for Pitta and promote general health. Melons are great for Pitta since they are cooling and hydrating, but they should be consumed alone. When prepared correctly, leafy greens such as spinach and kale balance the three doshas and are both nutritious and purifying. Beets, carrots, and squash are nutritious and grounding foods that are especially good for Vata and Pitta doshas.

In the Ayurvedic diet, dairy products—especially milk, yogurt, and ghee—have a unique role. As it provides all the necessary nutrients and fosters ojas, the life-giving energy that supports immunity, milk is regarded as a complete diet. To improve its digestion, it should be eaten warm and flavored with things like cardamom or ginger. When consumed in moderation and cooked correctly—as in the case of lassi, a diluted yogurt drink—yogurt is cooling and helpful for digestion. As was already noted, ghee is widely prized for its medicinal and digestive qualities.

In an Ayurvedic kitchen, herbs and herbal formulations are also essential ingredients. Among the most popular are holy basil (tulsi), neem, amla (Indian gooseberry), ashwagandha, and triphala. Holy basil is highly valued for its immune-stimulating and adaptogenic qualities. Neem is utilized for skin health and cleansing and is a potent detoxifier. Amla is a highly potent vitamin C source that enhances immunity and general well-being. Ashwagandha is an adaptogen that improves strength and endurance while assisting the body in managing stress. The three fruits that makeup Triphala—amla, haritaki, and bibhitaki—combine to provide a powerful cleanse and digestive support.

An Ayurvedic kitchen often consists of these basic components plus a variety of nuts, seeds, and sweeteners. Because of their nutritional advantages, almonds, sesame seeds, and flaxseeds are frequently utilized. Grounding and nutritious almonds are good for both Pitta and Vata energies. Rich in grounding and calcium, sesame seeds are good for both Kapha and Vata. Omega-3 fatty acids included in flaxseeds help improve digestive health, especially for Vata-type individuals. It is better to use natural sweeteners like dates, jaggery, and honey rather than refined sugar. Mineral-rich and aiding in digestion is jaggery. In Ayurveda, honey is used medicinally to balance Vata and Kapha. However, Pitta should use honey cautiously. When consumed in moderation, dates are healthy and revitalizing for all doshas.

In Ayurveda, meal preparation and consumption are just as essential as the ingredients. Important guidelines include seasonal adaptations, mindful eating, and appropriate food pairings. For food to be as nutritious and therapeutic as possible, it should be cooked with love and eaten in a calm setting. To minimize digestive issues, it is important to consume fruits apart from meals or avoid combining dairy with sour fruits. Seasonal adjustments refer to adjusting the diet to suit the changing seasons. For example, to maintain a dosha balance, one should consume warm foods in the winter and cooling foods in the summer.

In summary, an Ayurvedic kitchen is a haven of health-giving elements that enhance dosha balance and general well-being. An Ayurvedic diet's main components include grains like rice and barley, legumes like mung beans and lentils, oils like ghee and sesame oil, spices like ginger and turmeric, fruits, vegetables, dairy products, herbs, nuts, seeds, and natural sweeteners. These substances have been selected for their medicinal qualities in addition to their nutritional worth. Ayurveda's holistic approach places a strong emphasis on seasonal adaptations, mindful eating, and appropriate food pairings to maximize health. Achieving a harmonic balance of body, mind, and spirit through everyday living and adopting these basic elements and concepts can lead to vigorous health and long life.

Basic Ayurvedic cooking techniques (e.g., tempering spices, making ghee)

Ayurveda emphasizes nutrition and food for maintaining health and preventing illness. The cooking methods that not only improve food flavor and aroma but also reveal the medicinal properties of different components are essential to this strategy. To create meals that feed the body, mind, and soul, basic Ayurvedic culinary methods are needed. These techniques include tempering spices, producing ghee, and preparing herbal teas. This section delves further into these methods, emphasizing their importance and the advantages they offer to Ayurvedic cooking.

Tempering spices, also referred to as "tadka" or "chunk," is an essential method in Ayurvedic recipes. To increase the flavor and therapeutic benefits of spices, whole or ground spices are added to heated oil or ghee in a pan to release their essential oils. The volatile chemicals in the spices are extracted by the heated oil or ghee, increasing their potency and bioavailability. Curry leaves, cumin seeds, mustard seeds, fennel seeds, coriander seeds, turmeric, and asafoetida are among the often-used spices for tempering. The first step in the process is to heat the oil or ghee until it is hot enough but not smoking. Following that, the spices are added in a particular order, with the tougher spices—like cumin and mustard seeds—being put first since they take longer to release their flavors. Other spices like asafoetida and turmeric are added as the seeds begin to sputter and become fragrant. The cooked veggies, dals, or rice are topped with tempered spices, which immediately improves the dish's taste profile, digestibility, and medicinal properties.

Making clarified butter or ghee is another fundamental Ayurvedic culinary method. In Ayurveda, ghee is highly valued for its many health advantages, which include enhancing digestion, nourishing tissues, and boosting general vigor. To make ghee, gradually heat unsalted butter until the milk particles separate and settle to the bottom and the fluid evaporates. After that, the ghee—a transparent, golden liquid—is carefully separated and stored. This process not only extends the butter's shelf life and stability at high cooking temperatures but also eliminates lactose and casein, making it appropriate for people with dietary allergies to dairy. Ghee is regarded as tri-doshic, balancing the vata, pitta, and kapha doshas. It is utilized in many Ayurvedic treatments, including nasya (nasal administration) and abhyanga (oil massage), as well as in cooking and as a foundation for herbal formulations.

Known as "kashayams" or "kwaths," the production of herbal teas and decoctions is a crucial skill in Ayurvedic cookery. To extract the therapeutic compounds of herbs and spices, they are simmered in water to create these drinks. Herbal teas often contain ginger, turmeric, tulsi (holy basil), coriander, cumin, fennel, and cardamom. Herbal teas are made by adding herbs to boiling water and simmering them for a certain amount of time, which maximizes the extraction of their health-promoting chemicals. After that, the tea is filtered and served warm. These teas are designed to target particular health issues, such as promoting immunity, decreasing inflammation, easing mental stress, and enhancing digestion. For instance, turmeric, ginger, and tulsi may be used in an immune-boosting tea, while cumin, coriander, and fennel might be used in a tea that aids digestion. Making herbal teas is an easy but powerful method to bring the therapeutic benefits of Ayurvedic herbs and spices into your everyday routine.

Ayurveda advocates steaming as a mild cooking method for vegetables since it preserves their inherent tastes and nutrients. When food is cooked using steam produced by boiling water, vitamins, minerals, and phytonutrients that may be lost during other cooking techniques, such as boiling or frying, are retained. This approach has a softer texture and a calming, cooling impact, making it very useful for Vata and Pitta doshas. To improve the flavor and digestibility of steamed veggies, you may add some tempered spices or a drizzle of ghee to season them. Idlis, a popular South Indian breakfast dish made from fermented rice and lentil batter, are prepared by steaming. It is a light, healthy, and easily digestible meal.

Alternatively known as "yogic cooking," slow cooking is another method that fits with Ayurvedic principles. By cooking food at moderate temperatures over lengthy periods of time, this technique preserves the nutritional integrity of the components and lets them release their flavors gradually. Rice, mung beans, and spices combine to make the traditional Ayurvedic cuisine kichari, which is best prepared slowly. Because of its ease of digestion, nutritional balance, and simplicity, kichari is frequently included in Ayurvedic cleansing regimens. The therapeutic properties of the dish are enhanced by the slow cooking method, which results in a nutritious and grounded dinner that is appropriate for all doshas. Herbal oils and decoctions, which are essential to many Ayurvedic treatments and therapies, are also made by slow cooking.

An ancient Ayurvedic method for improving food's nutritional content and digestion is fermentation. Foods that have undergone fermentation are high in healthy microorganisms that enhance digestion and promote gut health. Yogurt, buttermilk, dosas (fermented rice and lentil crepes), kanji (fermented carrot or beetroot drink), and other fermented foods are commonly consumed in Ayurveda. By enabling natural bacteria and yeast to break down the starches and sugars in food, fermentation produces a tasty, acidic product that is high in probiotics, vitamins, and enzymes and more superficial to digest. Fermented foods, with their sour taste, help balance Vata and Kapha doshas. Those with a Pitta constitution should consume them in moderation.

In Ayurvedic cooking, sautéing, also known as "bhuna," is a fast and effective way to prepare grains, legumes, and vegetables. Using this technique, food is cooked over medium-high heat in a tiny amount of oil or ghee, frequently with spices added to improve taste and texture. Because it increases warmth and lowers moisture content, sautéing is suitable for Vata and Kapha doshas because it makes food lighter and more straightforward to digest. Remember to use cooling oils like coconut oil and reduce cooking time to prevent overheating, especially for Pitta dosha. To augment both the flavor profile and nutritional composition of sautéed dishes, consider incorporating subtle spices, fresh herbs, and a touch of lemon or lime.

Another Ayurvedic culinary method is baking, which may be used to make everything from bread and pastries to veggies and grains. Baking preserves moisture and develops rich tastes in food by heating it in a confined space with dry heat. According to Ayurveda, baking is good for the Kapha dosha because it makes food lighter and easier to digest by reducing its heavy, wet texture. It's critical to utilize whole grain flour, natural sweets like jaggery or honey, and healthy fats like ghee or coconut oil in baked products to make sure they adhere to Ayurvedic principles. Warming spices like cardamom, ginger, and cinnamon can be added to baked foods to increase their medicinal benefits.

Apart from these methods of cooking, Ayurveda also emphasizes the need to carefully prepare and consume food. It is said that cooking with intention and good energy imbues the food with prana, or life force, amplifying its nourishing and restorative qualities. For best digestion and nutritional absorption, meals should be prepared in a tidy, peaceful setting and eaten in a quiet, relaxed way. Appropriate pairings of foods, such as avoiding sour fruits and milk or eating fruits apart from meals, are crucial for preventing upset stomachs and improving the body's absorption of nutrients.

To sum up, fundamental Ayurvedic culinary methods, including blending ghee, tempering spices, brewing herbal teas, steaming, slow cooking, fermenting, sautéing, and baking, are essential for producing dishes that are healthy for the body, mind, and soul. These methods assist the equilibrium of the doshas and general well-being by enhancing the flavor and scent of food as well as revealing the medicinal properties of diverse components. Ayurveda's holistic approach places a strong emphasis on using seasonal and locally sourced foods, preparing and consuming meals mindfully, and creating appropriate food combinations. Achieving a harmonic balance of body, mind, and spirit by daily application of these practices and ideas can result in vigorous health and long life. The ageless knowledge of Ayurvedic cookery provides a road to well-being that is profoundly applicable in the modern world while still having solid roots in tradition.

CHAPTER IV

Recipes for Vata Balance

Warm porridges and nourishing smoothies

Warm porridges and filling smoothies have gained popularity in contemporary diets because of their pleasant qualities, adaptability, and health advantages. These recipes are perfect for every meal of the day because they provide a special blend of warmth, nourishment, and enjoyment. This section explores the origins, health advantages, and cooking techniques of warm porridges and filling smoothies, emphasizing their significance in today's health-conscious society.

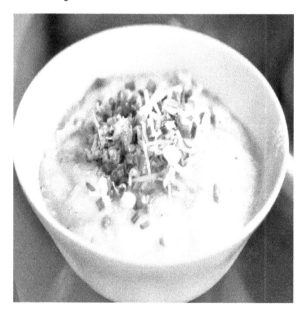

The history of porridge extends back to prehistoric times. Grain varieties, including barley, oats, and millet, were used to make the first porridges, which were boiled in milk or water until they were thick and creamy. Porridge has long been a staple meal and is frequently connected to comfort and nourishment in a variety of cultures. For instance, oatmeal porridge is a common morning food in Scotland and is typically eaten with honey or a touch of salt. Rice porridge, known as congee, is a popular morning food in China. It can occasionally be seasoned with meat, vegetables, or preserved eggs.

Conversely, smoothies are very new, having first appeared in the middle of the 20th century when electric blenders became available. Smoothies acquired popularity among fitness enthusiasts and in health food stores at first, but their convenience and nutritional value rapidly made them popular among the general public. A range of nutrients could be easily consumed in a single dose because of the smooth, drinkable form that was created by combining fruits, vegetables, and other components. Smoothies have become a worldwide trend in recent times, with many versions to suit a variety of palates and dietary requirements.

Rich smoothies and warm porridge are both packed with nourishment and are great options for a well-rounded diet. Usually cooked from whole grains, porridge is a great way to get fiber, complex carbs, and important vitamins and minerals. For instance, oats have a sizable quantity of soluble fiber that dissolves in water, which lowers cholesterol and helps to control blood sugar. Important elements, including iron, magnesium, and B vitamins, are also present in them. Another excellent source of calcium and protein is oatmeal, especially when cooked with milk or fortified plant-based substitutes.

Smoothies, on the other hand, are packed with nutrients because of how many fruits and vegetables they include. Because these nutrients are high in mineral content, vitamins, antioxidants, and fiber, they support overall health and well-being. A smoothie including spinach, bananas, and berries, for instance, offers a substantial amount of potassium, vitamin C, and dietary fiber in addition to healthful phytochemicals. Smoothies may be made more protein-dense by adding items like yogurt, nut butter, or protein powder. This makes them a fulfilling and well-balanced lunch alternative.

Making warm porridges and filling smoothies is a great way to express your creativity and meet a variety of dietary needs and nutritional objectives.

Start with a grain foundation, such as quinoa, rice, or oats, to produce a simple porridge. In a pot, mix the grains with a liquid (milk, water, or plant-based substitute). If the mixture reaches a boil, reduce the heat and continue cooking the cooked porridge until the required consistency and softness of the grains are achieved. You can experiment with the liquid-to-grain ratio to suit your tastes; a higher liquid content will provide a creamier porridge. Porridge may be improved by adding a wide range of mix-ins and toppings, including nuts, seeds, dried or fresh fruit, spices, and sweeteners, once it has been prepared. For instance, sliced bananas, cinnamon, and maple syrup drizzled over a bowl of oatmeal porridge make a tasty and nourishing breakfast.

Smoothies are simple to make and just as adaptable. Start with a liquid foundation, such as milk, juice, or water, then top with a variety of fruits and vegetables. Avocado, kale, spinach, berries, and bananas are often used components in smoothies. Try adding protein powder, silken tofu, or yogurt for more creaminess and protein. Blend the ingredients until they are combined, adding or eliminating liquid as needed to get the desired consistency. Superfoods and supplements, including chia seeds, flaxseeds, spirulina, or matcha powder, can be added to smoothies to further personalize them. For example, a green smoothie with Greek yogurt, spinach, kiwi, and a teaspoon of spirulina is not only nutrient-dense but also colorful and energizing.

Including nutritious smoothies and warm porridges in your regular diet can have a big impact on your health. These foods are high in nutrients, which promote heart health and healthy digestion, among other elements of well-being. Smoothies' and porridges' high fiber content encourages regularity and a healthy digestive system, which helps to ward against constipation and maintain a balanced gut flora. Antioxidant substances discovered in agricultural products can aid in the battle against discomfort and cellular oxidative stress, two diseases associated with long-term conditions, which includes cancer as well as cardiovascular disease.

These meals also support healthy weight management. Porridge's fiber and complex carbs provide you with a sensation of fullness and lasting energy, which might help you avoid overindulging. Similar to this, smoothies' high nutritional density makes them a filling supper choice that can reduce unhealthy snacking. People may enjoy varied and well-balanced meals that promote their overall health objectives by including a range of fruits, vegetables, and other nutrient-dense products.

Ecological and moral principles can also be considered while selecting components for smoothies and porridges. Choosing seasonal, organic, and locally grown foods lessens the environmental effect of food production and delivery. To make these recipes vegan-friendly and less dependent on animal products, try using plant-based milk substitutes like oats, soy, or almond milk. This will help to create a more sustainable food system.

Smoothies and porridges are great ways to use up overripe fruits and leftover veggies if you're trying to reduce food waste. Too-soft bananas can be frozen and used in smoothies to provide a naturally sweet and creamy texture. Vegetable leftovers may also be preserved and blended into smoothies to give extra nutrition and reduce waste.

Comfort, nutrition, and variety are all provided by warming porridges and filling smoothies, which are the ideal fusion of tradition and contemporary. Their versatility and nutritional advantages make them perfect for today's health-conscious lives, and their rich history and cultural importance only serve to highlight their timeless appeal. People who are aware of the cooking techniques and the health benefits of these healthful foods can readily include them in their daily routines and reap the many benefits they provide. Whether you want to fuel up with a nutrient-dense smoothie in the morning or start the day with a warm bowl of porridge, these meals offer a tasty and fulfilling method to boost general health and well-being.

Grounding soups and stews

Soups and stews that are grounding have long been a mainstay of many culinary traditions worldwide, valued for their capacity to balance and feed the body in addition to their soothing tastes. These filling foods are notably valued in Ayurveda, the age-old Indian holistic medicine system, for their capacity to balance and root the doshas, particularly Vata. This section examines the idea of "grounding foods," discusses the health and nutritional advantages of soups and stews, and provides tips on how to cook these meals to bring out their most grounding and healing qualities.

According to Ayurvedic philosophy, meals that balance the vata dosha's light, airy, and mobile properties are considered grounding foods. Vata controls communication and mobility throughout the body and is made up of the elements of air and space. Vata gives vibrancy, inventiveness, and flexibility when it is in balance. On the other hand, when it is out of balance, it can cause stomach problems, anxiety, and restlessness. Warm, wet, heavy, and nourishing dishes are often considered grounding foods since they serve to balance and soothe Vata's volatile character.

Many of these balancing traits are seen in soups and stews, which are classic grounding meals. The fact that they are often served warm helps to soothe Vata's chilly disposition. Maintaining the Vata balance requires breaking down the fibers in meats and vegetables through cooking, which facilitates digestion. These foods' moisture content balances out Vata's natural tendency toward dryness by giving the body's tissues the vital water and lubrication they need.

Soups and stews are nutritious powerhouses full of vitamins, minerals, and macronutrients. They frequently have a diverse range of proteins, legumes, and vegetables, providing a well-rounded nutritional profile. Carrots, potatoes, and leafy greens, for instance, are high in vitamins A, C, and K and high in vital minerals like magnesium and potassium. These ingredients may also be found in a traditional vegetable stew. Legumes, such as beans or lentils, increase the protein level of a food, making it more filling and supplying energy for longer. Meats offer more protein, iron, and B vitamins, all of which are essential for sustaining energy generation, muscular growth, and general health.

Soups and stews benefit from the slow-cooking method because it increases the nutrients' bioavailability, which facilitates the body's absorption and utilization. Vegetable cell walls are broken down during cooking, releasing nutrients that could otherwise be kept inside. This procedure also helps the flavors to combine, resulting in a wonderful and nutrient-dense rich and comforting meal.

Using warming herbs and spices is one of the main elements of grounding soups and stews. Spices like ginger, turmeric, cumin, and coriander are frequently used in Ayurvedic cookery to strengthen the digestive fire or Agni. For nutrients to be properly broken down and assimilated, the digestive fire must be powerful. For example, ginger is a great ingredient in soups and stews for those with Vata imbalances because of its anti-inflammatory and digestive qualities. In addition to adding a striking color, turmeric's strong anti-inflammatory and antioxidant qualities also promote general health and well-being.

Adding healthy fats to soups and stews is another crucial step in grounding them. Because they create a feeling of fullness and slow down digestion—which is advantageous for Vata types who could have irregular digestion—fats are essential for anchoring. Soups and stews that contain ghee, coconut oil, or olive oil can become more grounding and help absorb fat-soluble vitamins (A, D, E, and K). In Ayurveda, ghee, or clarified butter, is especially valued for its capacity to support both the body and the mind and for giving food a rich, buttery flavor.

To make soups and stews more grounded, you may also add grains like barley, quinoa, and rice. For instance, the high fiber content of brown rice and millet helps to maintain constant blood sugar levels and a healthy digestive system. Since quinoa is a complete protein—that is, it includes all nine essential amino acids—it is an excellent supplement for anybody attempting to improve their protein intake.

Another essential ingredient for earthy soups and stews is root vegetables. In addition to being high in nutrients, vegetables like sweet potatoes, carrots, and beets also offer a calming, naturally sweet flavor. Carrots are a wonderful source of fiber, antioxidants, and vitamins A and K; sweet potatoes are high in beta-carotene, potassium, and vitamin C. In addition to being rich in nitrates, manganese, and folate—all of which promote cardiovascular health—beets are also well-known for their cleansing qualities.

Black beans, lentils, and chickpeas are examples of legumes that are frequently used in soups and stews to provide both fiber and protein. Specifically, lentils are an excellent source of iron, folate, and plant-based protein, making them a nutrient-dense complement to any meal. Because they are high in protein and fiber, chickpeas can help to balance blood sugar levels and prolong feelings of fullness. In addition to adding a substantial texture to soups and stews, black beans are a great source of vitamins, minerals, and antioxidants.

Making grounded stews and soups requires careful attention to detail in the kitchen. Eating food that has been carefully and intentionally prepared can enhance its therapeutic effects by adding positive energy to the dish. According to Ayurveda, cooking is a type of meditation in which the emotions and mental state of the chef can affect the finished product. A more wholesome and fulfilling dinner may be produced when cooking with love, gratitude, and awareness.

A common foundation soup in Ayurvedic cooking is called kitchari, a straightforward yet hearty dish prepared with rice and mung beans that is flavored with coriander, cumin, and turmeric. Because kitchari is simple to digest and offers a complete diet, it is frequently used in Ayurvedic cleaning regimens. The spices aid in digestion and cleansing, and the mix of rice and mung beans yields a complete protein. Kitchari may be tailored to each person's preferences and dosha requirements by adding different veggies and herbs.

Moroccan Harira is a classic soup composed of lentils, chickpeas, tomatoes, and a combination of warming spices like cumin, cinnamon, and ginger. It's another well-liked stew that acts as a grounding agent. Harira is a filling and substantial dish that is frequently given during Ramadan to break the fast. Legumes, veggies, and spices work together to create a well-balanced meal that aids in digestion and gives you energy again.

Beef stew is a traditional example of a grounding meal in Western cuisine. Meat stew is made with pieces of meat, fragrant herbs, and root vegetables that are simmered gently to create rich, deep tastes. The broth gets a gelatinous texture from the collagen in the cattle bones, which is good for digestion and joint health. Because of its substantial texture, beef stew is the ideal comfort dish for chilly weather, offering warmth and nourishment.

The meal known as "Jewish penicillin," or chicken soup, is another nourishing and calming one. When feeling under the weather, chicken soup, which is cooked with chicken, vegetables, and herbs, is often consumed. It is said to have immune-boosting qualities. The broth's high mineral and gelatin content promotes hydration and digestive health. The soup's grounding properties are strengthened with the addition of root vegetables like carrots and parsnips, which make it nutritious and soothing.

Lentil stew and butternut squash soup are two examples of vegetarian dishes that are filling and healthy. The creamy and cozy texture of butternut squash soup is achieved by combining roasted squash, onions, and a small amount of nutmeg. Squash is a nutrient-dense food that is high in fiber, antioxidants, and vitamins A and C. A satisfying and high-protein dinner may be had with lentil stew, which is prepared using lentils, tomatoes, and a variety of veggies. Legumes and veggies work well together to provide a filling, well-balanced meal that improves digestion and general health.

In conclusion, especially when considering Ayurveda, hearty soups and stews are an essential element of a well-rounded and healthy diet. Warmth, wetness, and nutrients are provided by these foods, which aid in body and mind stabilization and relaxation. A well-rounded nutritional profile is ensured by including a range of vegetables, legumes, proteins, and healthy fats. Additionally, the therapeutic effects of these foods are enhanced by the use of warming spices and attentive cooking techniques. Grounded soups and stews are a tasty and fulfilling way to nurture your body and spirit, whether your goals are balance, comfort, or improved health.

Hearty grains and root vegetables

For millennia, wholesome grains and root vegetables have been mainstays of diets in several societies over the globe, praised for their nutritive worth, adaptability, and capacity to offer prolonged vitality. These foods serve as the foundation of many traditional diets and provide a host of health advantages, such as better digestion, increased nutritional intake, and support for general well-being. This section explores the nutritional characteristics, health advantages, culinary applications, and cultural significance of robust grains and root vegetables.

Hearty grains are prized for their complex carbohydrate content, which releases energy gradually and steadily, promoting stable blood sugar levels and extending satiety. Examples of these grains are barley, quinoa, brown rice, millet, and farro. For instance, barley is a complete grain that has been farmed for more than 10,000 years. It offers a lot of fiber, especially beta-glucan, which has been demonstrated to decrease cholesterol and strengthen heart health. Important vitamins and minerals found in barley include iron, magnesium, selenium, and B vitamins. It works well as an ingredient in salads, soups, stews, and side dishes because of its chewy texture and nutty flavor.

Although quinoa is actually a seed and is sometimes categorized as a grain because of its comparable culinary applications, it is more widely known as a superfood. Quinoa, which comes from South America's Andes, is a complete protein because it has all nine necessary amino acids, which the body is unable to manufacture on its own. Because of this, it's a great source of protein for vegans and vegetarians. In addition, quinoa has a lot of fiber, antioxidants, and important minerals, including magnesium, phosphorus, manganese, and folate. It may be used in a variety of recipes, from savory salads and main meals to breakfast porridge, thanks to its mild flavor and fluffy texture.

Another whole grain that is popularly consumed worldwide is brown rice. Brown rice, in contrast to white rice, keeps its fiber- vitamin- and mineral-rich bran and germ layers. Because of this, brown rice is a more nutrient-dense choice and a rich source of magnesium, manganese, selenium, and B vitamins. Because brown rice has so much fiber, it improves gut microbiota health, facilitates digestion, and helps control weight by making you feel fuller for longer. It's somewhat chewy texture and nutty flavor go well with stir-fries, pilaf's, and grain bowls, among other things.

Asia and Africa are the two regions where millet is most common. It is an ancient grain that has been farmed for thousands of years. This grain is extremely nutrient-dense, having high levels of fiber, protein, and important minerals, including manganese, phosphorus, and magnesium. In addition, those with gluten-in or gluten sensitivity can eat millet, which is a crop that is devoid of gluten. It may be used in savory and sweet recipes, such as bread, salads, and casseroles, because of its mild, somewhat sweet flavor.

For ages, the ancient wheat grain known as farro has been a mainstay in Mediterranean cuisine. It is well-known for both its outstanding nutritional profile and nutty taste and chewy texture. High in fiber, protein, and important minerals like iron, zinc, and magnesium, farro is a nutritious food. Farro's high fiber content aids in blood sugar stabilization, digestive regulation, and heart health promotion. Because of its substantial texture, it works well in salads, soups, and grain bowls to create filling and healthy meals.

Carrots, sweet potatoes, beets, turnips, and parsnips are examples of root vegetables. These are subterranean plant sections that are high in bioactive chemicals and important nutrients. Carrots, for example, are an excellent retailer of the pigment beta-car, which the body utilizes to produce the antioxidant vitamin A that is essential for strong immune systems, healthy skin, and eyes. Moreover, they contain a lot of fiber, which promotes digestive health and a healthy weight. Carrots are a versatile element in both raw and cooked recipes, from salads and snacks to soups and stews, because of their sweet flavor and crisp texture.

Another nutrient-dense root vegetable with a bright orange hue and inherent sweetness is sweet potatoes. Beta-carotene, vitamin C, potassium, and fiber are abundant in them. Sweet potatoes have a high antioxidant content that helps shield the body from inflammation and oxidative damage. They are a well-liked option for many different foods, such as casseroles, fries, soups, and desserts, because of their inherent sweetness and creamy texture.

Beets are vibrant red or golden vegetables that are rich in important minerals and antioxidants. They are a great source of potassium, manganese, dietary nitrates, and folate. It has been demonstrated that the nitrates in beets increase blood flow, decrease blood pressure, and improve athletic performance. Beets are a flexible addition to salads, drinks, soups, and roasted vegetable medleys because of their earthy taste and bright color.

Turnips are a nutrient-dense and adaptable root vegetable that is sometimes disregarded in contemporary diets. They are low in calories but high in the nutrient's potassium, fiber, and vitamin C. Moreover, turnips contain substances called compounds, which have anti-cancer qualities. They work well for mashing, roasting, and adding to soups and stews because of their firm texture and somewhat peppery taste.

Parsnips resemble carrots in appearance and taste sweet and nutty. They are high in potassium, folate, fiber, and vitamins C and K. Parsnips' fiber facilitates digestion, and their vitamins and minerals promote general health and well-being. Parsnips are a filling and healthy complement to any meal, whether they are roasted, mashed, or added to soups and stews.

Eating a diet high in whole grains and root vegetables has several health advantages. These foods are high in fiber, promoting regular bowel movements and preventing constipation, thus improving digestive health. In addition, fiber is critical for preserving a balanced gut flora, which is critical for immunological and general health. Furthermore, the natural sugars in root vegetables and complex carbs in grains offer a consistent energy supply that avoids blood sugar troughs and surges.

Grains and root vegetables include vitamins and minerals that assist a number of body processes, including the synthesis of energy, immune system support, bone health, and muscular function. For instance, the potassium in root vegetables maintains heart health and muscular function, while the B vitamins in grains aid in the conversion of food into energy. These foods' antioxidants lower the body's vulnerability to oxidative stress and inflammation, which lowers the likelihood of developing chronic illnesses, including cancer, diabetes, and heart disease.

Global culinary customs honor the adaptability and nutritive worth of substantial grains and root crops. Farro is commonly used in Italian cooking for its chewy texture and nutty flavor, often found in soups and salads. A traditional recipe is farro salad with roasted vegetables, which consists of farro mixed with roasted beets, carrots, and parsnips and topped with balsamic vinegar and olive oil. This delightful dish not only excites the taste buds with its delicious flavors, but it also provides a generous number of antioxidants to help support overall health. Furthermore, it's loaded with crucial vitamins and fiber, making it a wholesome and fulfilling option for a meal.

Grains and root vegetables are staples in many Indian recipes. A well-liked cuisine is khichdi, a hearty and nourishing dish composed of rice, lentils, and a variety of vegetables, including turnips, carrots, and sweet potatoes. Ginger, cumin, and turmeric provide flavor to khichdi, which is simple to digest and a well-balanced meal that promotes general health. The aromatic curry known as "aloo gobi," which is cooked with potatoes, cauliflower, and a mixture of spices, is another popular meal. This recipe demonstrates how adaptable root vegetables are and how well they take on and balance a variety of tastes.

Root vegetables like burdock root and daikon radish are frequently used in soups and stews in Japanese cooking. Oden, a filling stew cooked in a soy-based broth with daikon, tofu, boiled eggs, and different fish cakes, is one of the most well-liked dishes. Oden's root vegetables take up the flavors of the broth, making for a filling and healthy supper. Daikon radish's crisp texture and spicy flavor make it a popular addition to pickles and salads.

Millet and root vegetables are the main ingredients in many traditional African cuisines. Fufu is one such starchy side dish that goes well with soups and stews. It is created from mashed yams or cassava. For rich and delicious recipes like groundnut stew, which is cooked with peanuts, sweet potatoes, and leafy greens, fufu makes a dense and hearty basis. Jollof rice is a popular single-pot meal made with rice, tomatoes, and assorted vegetables. Jollof rice's blend of grains and veggies makes for a wholesome and well-balanced dinner.

Quinoa and root vegetables are prized for their nutritious content and adaptability in South American cooking. Quinoa soup, prepared with quinoa, potatoes, carrots, and a blend of spices, is a classic meal. This comforting, hearty soup offers all the necessary elements along with a comprehensive dose of protein. Roasted root vegetable medley is another well-liked recipe that combines the flavors and color of roasted sweet potatoes, beets, and carrots with olive oil and herbs to make a tasty and vibrant side dish.

Beyond their nutritional worth, robust cereals and root vegetables have cultural importance. These meals are essential to many religious and cultural traditions and also have symbolic importance. Grains are seen as fertility and plenty symbols in many civilizations. For instance, rice is frequently utilized in religious rites and festivities and is revered in many Asian civilizations. Grains like sorghum and millet are employed in ceremonies and community feasts in African societies, where they are symbolic of wealth.

Root-based crops additionally hold symbolic importance in many civilizations. In keeping with Celtic tradition, root veggies like turnip greens and beets have been cut into lanterns for the Samhain ceremony, which marks the close of the crop-growing season and the beginning of winter. Eventually, this custom gave rise to the Halloween pumpkin-carving ritual that exists today. Daikon radish is featured in many New Year's meals in Japanese culture as a sign of longevity and good fortune. Root vegetables are an essential component of many traditional rites and festivities because of their vivid colors and anchoring attributes.

Hearty grains and root vegetables are becoming more and more important components of modern diets because of their sustainability and health advantages. When compared to animal-based goods, these meals are frequently more economical and ecologically beneficial, making them a sustainable option for people and the environment. Traditional grains and root vegetables are seeing a rebirth in popularity as plant-based diets gain traction. Home cooks and professional chefs are exploring innovative ways to incorporate these ingredients into their dishes.

In summary, a diet rich in nutrients and balance must include both robust grains and root vegetables. They provide several health advantages, such as better digestion, long-lasting energy, and support for general well-being. They are essential to many culinary traditions worldwide because of their adaptability and cultural importance. You may respect their cultural legacy and promote sustainable food practices while savoring the mouthwatering tastes, rich textures, and countless health advantages of a diverse range of grains and root vegetables.

Herbal teas and snacks to soothe Vata

Ayurveda, the age-old Indian holistic medical system, heavily relies on herbal teas and snacks, especially when it comes to balancing the three doshas of Pitta, Kapha, and Vata. Different physiological traits and functions correlate with each dosha. Vata is the element of air and space; it governs the neurological system, movement, and communication. Vata encourages vitality, inventiveness, and flexibility when it is in balance. On the other hand, too much Vata can cause problems, including anxiety, restlessness, dry skin, constipation, and insomnia. It is crucial to include warming, nutritious, and grounding meals and beverages to offset these effects. This section examines several herbal teas and snacks that are intended to balance and calm the Vata dosha, with a focus on the components, methods of preparation, and health advantages of each.

A potent and calming treatment for reducing Vata dosha is herbal tea. Vata is chilly, dry, and unpredictable; teas created from warming, grounding, and relaxing herbs can help balance it. Ginger is one of the best herbs for Vata dosha. The warming qualities of ginger tea, which is brewed from fresh ginger root, are well known. It aids in reducing inflammation, enhancing circulation, and promoting digestion. Ginger tea is a warming beverage that tastes strong and slightly sweet, especially in the winter. Simmer fresh ginger root slices in water for ten to fifteen minutes to make ginger tea. Its calming benefits can be further enhanced by adding a small amount of honey.

Licorice root tea is another herbal beverage that works well for Vata. Licorice root is well-known for both its tasty flavor and its stress-relieving, adaptogenic qualities. It is also perfect for alleviating Vata's dry and unpredictable tendencies because of its anti-inflammatory and demulcent (soothing) properties on the digestive tract. To create licorice root tea, steep powdered fennel root with a pot of water until approximately ten minutes. Licorice root can cause hypertension if taken in excess; therefore, it's vital to remember that it should be used sparingly, especially for people with high blood pressure.

Another great option for calming Vata is chamomile tea. Because of its gentle, sedative qualities, chamomile helps relax and soothe the nervous system. It is especially helpful in treating digestive disorders, anxiety, and insomnia—all of which are frequently brought on by a

Vata imbalance. To create chamomile tea, soak dried chamomile flowers in simmering water approximately five to ten minutes. You may enhance its calming and warming effects by adding a small teaspoon of cinnamon.

Ayurveda places great value on ashwagandha tea, which is brewed from the plant's root and has adaptogenic and grounding qualities. Ashwagandha promotes general well-being, increases energy, and lowers stress. It works very well to balance the Vata dosha by enhancing mental acuity and physical vigor. Simmer ashwagandha root powder in water for ten to fifteen minutes to prepare ashwagandha tea. It can have more flavor and calming effects if a tiny amountof milk and a sweetener like jaggery or honey are added.

Another useful choice for regulating Vata is cardamom tea. Warming cardamom improves circulation, soothes the nervous system, and helps with digestion. To create cardamom tea, crush a handful of cardamom pods and soak them in simmering water to obtain around ten minutes. Cardamom can be used with other spices, such as ginger and cinnamon, to make a flavorful and cozy mixture.

Tulsi, sometimes referred to as divine basil, is highly prized in Ayurveda for its numerous health benefits. The well-known adaptogenic qualities of Tulasi tea support the body's ability to stay balanced and adjust to stress. Moreover, it possesses antioxidant, antibacterial, and anti-inflammatory properties. Tea made from Tulsi leaves is especially good for reducing Vata dosha since it boosts immunity, calms the nervous system, and improves mental clarity. Steep dried tulsi leaves in boiling water for five to ten minutes in order to make tulsi tea. Its flavor can be improved by sprinkling in some honey or lemon.

Snacks are just as vital as herbal teas in balancing the Vata dosha. Vata types benefit from warm, moist, nourishing snacks that provide stability and nourishment.

Warm spiced milk is one of the best snacks for Vata dosha. Since milk is naturally nutritious and grounding, it becomes even more helpful when paired with warming spices. Warm up a cup of milk, then add a dash of cardamom, nutmeg, and cinnamon to make spiced milk. Its calming effects can be amplified by adding a sweetener like jaggery or honey. This beverage is especially helpful right before bed because it encourages unwinding and peaceful sleep.

Another great snack to help calm Vata is oatmeal. Oats are a naturally nutritious and grounding food that offers stability and long-lasting energy. Oatmeal can be made more Vata-pacifying by heating the milk and adding warming spices like nutmeg and cinnamon. To add even more nutrition and taste, you can mix in a handful of nuts and dried fruits.

Vata is also benefited by cooked fruits, such as stewed apples or pears. Fruits that have been cooked are easier to digest and help counteract the dry and light characteristics of Vata. Peel and cut apples or pears, then cook them in a tiny amount of water with spices such as ginger, cloves, and cinnamon to make stewed fruits. They can be made sweeter with a maple syrup or honey to enhance the flavor and relaxing effects.

Beets, carrots, and sweet potatoes are examples of root vegetables that are great as snacks to help ground Vata. These vegetables offer vital vitamins and minerals and are naturally delicious and nutritious. The flavor and Vata-pacifying qualities of root vegetables can be improved by roasting or steam-charging them with warming spices such as turmeric, coriander, and cumin. They can be served with olive oil or ghee to intensify their grounding properties.

Nuts and seeds are good snacks for Vata as well. Sesame seeds, walnuts, and almonds are especially nourishing and grounding. Nuts can be healthier for Vata and easier to digest if soaked overnight. Nuts and dried fruits such as figs, raisins, and dates can be combined to make a tasty and filling snack that gives you energy and sustenance all day long.

Vata is especially benefiting from sesame seed treats like sesame seed balls or brittle. Rich in calcium, magnesium, and healthy fats, sesame seeds support and balance Vata. Toast the sesame seeds and mix them with honey or melted jaggery to make the sesame seeds brittle. Before dividing the mixture into pieces, press it onto a level surface and allow it to cool. Til ladoo, or roasted sesame balls, are produced by combining roasted sesame seeds with honey or jaggery and forming the mixture into little balls. Not only are these snacks tasty, but they also offer prolonged energy and nutrients.

Ghee-roasted nuts are a useful snack for Vata dosha as well. In Ayurveda, ghee, or clarified butter, is highly valued for its nourishing and anchoring qualities. A tasty and balanced snack can be made by roasting nuts like walnuts, cashews, or almonds in ghee and adding some salt and spices like cinnamon or cumin. Nuts roasted in ghee offer vital nutrients, protein, and good fats that balance vata.

It's also possible to combine herbal teas and munchies to make calming and filling meals. For instance, black tea, milk, and a mixture of warming spices like ginger, cardamom, cinnamon, and cloves can be used to make chai tea, a classic Indian spiced tea. Chai tea is a great option for Vata because it is naturally calming and grounding. Chai tea served with sesame seed snacks or nuts roasted in ghee is a comprehensive and filling Vata-pacifying treat.

Herbal drinks and snacks might be a great way to balance and calm the Vata dosha in your everyday routine. It is crucial to eat and drink these meals and beverages carefully, considering personal tastes and portion sizes.

Enhancing the efficiency of these medicines can be achieved by paying attention to the body's needs and modifying them according to the seasons and individual constitution.

Apart from dietary modifications, lifestyle choices can also be very important for maintaining Vata balance. Establishing consistent daily habits, including getting up and going to bed at the same time, might help balance Vata's unpredictable tendencies. Walking, tai chi, and yoga are examples of gentle activities that can assist in grounding and calming Vata. Calming the nerves and promoting serenity can also be achieved through the practice of deep respiration and other mindfulness practices.

Furnishing a cozy and welcoming home might help maintain Vata's equilibrium even more. A tranquil environment can be produced by keeping the house warm, utilizing soft and cuddly textiles, and adding soothing hues like earthy tones. In addition to promoting relaxation and calming Vata, aromatherapy using essential oils like frankincense, sandalwood, and lavender can also aid.

To sum up, herbal teas and snacks are essential for calming and achieving a balanced Vata dosha. Vata is characterized by coldness, dryness, and erraticness. Warming, grounding, and nourishing meals and drinks can assist to counteract these attributes and promote stability, relaxation, and general well-being. Herbal teas made with licorice root, cardamom, tulsi, ginger, chamomile, and ashwagandha are easy when incorporating into everyday activities and offer a host of health benefits. Nuts, seeds, cooked fruits, root vegetables, oats, flavored milk, and other snacks supply vital nutrition and balance Vata. By integrating these dietary adjustments with conscious lifestyle choices, Vata balance, and optimum health can be achieved holistically.

People can attain more peace and well-being in their lives by comprehending and adhering to the principles of Ayurveda.

CHAPTER V

Mindful Eating Practices

Setting up your dining space

Creating an atmosphere that improves the dining experience, encourages comfort, and represents individual taste and practicality goes beyond just putting furniture in its proper place. A thoughtfully planned eating space can make meals become special occasions that promote happiness and connection. This section will look at the essential elements of creating a dining room, such as selecting the right lighting and furniture and considering the layout, style, and ambiance. Any dining area's central feature is the dining table. The size of the room, the average number of diners, the design and material of the table, and other factors all need to be considered when selecting a table. Rectangular tables offer enough seats for bigger groups and fit nicely in the majority of dining rooms. However, because they face each other, round tables are perfect for compact areas and encourage intimacy and conversation. Square tables fit well in both small and medium-sized settings and have a contemporary appearance. Another important consideration is the type of material used for the table; metal tables provide an industrial, sleek appearance, glass tables offer a contemporary touch and give the impression of space, and hardwood tables radiate warmth and heritage.

Dining chair selection is equally crucial. Comfort is crucial because visitors should be relaxed while eating. Chairs with upholstery provide comfort and suppleness, which makes them perfect for extended dining sessions. But compared to metal or wooden chairs, which are more resilient and easier to clean, they need more upkeep. The chairs' height and design have to go well with the table and the general look of the space. Larger dining rooms are the ideal fit for chairs with armrests since they enhance comfort without sacrificing space.

The eating area's flow and usefulness are greatly impacted by its layout. The dining area in an open-plan house should be able to blend in with the kitchen and living areas without losing its own character. The dining experience can be improved by positioning the dining table close to a window, which lets in natural light and provides a pleasant view. It's important to make sure there's adequate room around the table for comfortable mobility; ideally, the table should be at least 36 inches away from any walls or other furniture. This makes it possible for visitors to move around comfortably and sit down.

Setting the tone and atmosphere of the eating area is largely dependent on the lighting. An attractive ambiance is created by combining task, ambient, and accent lighting. Above the dining table, chandeliers or pendant lights create a decorative focal point and direct, focused lighting. It's crucial to choose the right height for these lights; they should be low enough to foster intimacy but high enough to prevent getting in the way of views and talks. Dimmer switches provide versatility by enabling the light's intensity to be changed based on the situation, such as a formal gathering or a laid-back family meal.

Wall sconces and floor lights can provide layers of light and create a warm, pleasant ambiance in addition to overhead lighting. Another great method to improve the atmosphere is with candles, which provide a mellow, flickering illumination that encourages unwinding and discussion. The sort of bulbs used can also have an impact on the mood; colder white bulbs produce a more contemporary, upbeat air, while warm white lighting creates a feeling of coziness and invitingness.

The dining room's color scheme and décor selections establish the mood and showcase individual preferences. Furniture and décor items can stand out against a timeless and elegant backdrop created by neutral colors like beige, white, and gray. Vibrant hues like rich blues, greens, or reds can provide warmth and drama while still creating a homey, personal sense in the dining room. Mirrors, artwork, and wallpaper are great ways to add patterns and textures to a room, giving it visual interest and character.

The way that tables are set up and linens are used greatly influences the whole dining experience. Good tableware, such as glasses, plates, and silverware, improves the visual attractiveness of the table in addition to its practical use. A harmonious appearance is produced by coordinating these pieces with the room's general color scheme and design. Table linens, which include napkins, runners, and tablecloths, give a touch of refinement and elegance. It makes sense to choose textiles that are simple to keep clean and maintain, especially for regular use. The dining area may be kept feeling new and inviting all year long with seasonal adjustments to the table arrangements and linens.

Having storage options is crucial to keeping your eating area tidy. Tableware, linens, and other dining necessities can be stored in buffets, sideboards, and cabinets to keep them neat and handy. Additionally, these furniture pieces provide more surface area for serving food and beverages during events. A harmonious and well-coordinated design can be achieved by choosing storage pieces whose style and substance suit those of the dining table and chairs.

Adding natural materials to the dining area can improve its aesthetics and foster a calm atmosphere. A touch of organic beauty and coziness is added by using natural materials like wood and stone, fresh flowers, and potted plants. Seasonal floral or greenery centerpieces can be changed out with the seasons to keep the dining room interesting and vibrant. A cozy, welcoming ambiance can also be produced by using natural fibers in curtains, rugs, and tablecloths.

The requirements and lifestyles of the users should also be reflected in the dining area. Durability and cleaning convenience are crucial factors to consider for households with little children. Even with frequent usage, the room will stay stylish and useful thanks to sturdy furniture and machine-washable textiles. A bigger table with movable leaves and more seating options can easily fit guests for people who party frequently. Versatility is increased in the area with multipurpose furniture, such as benches that serve as both seating and storage.

Although they are frequently disregarded, acoustic factors are quite important to the dining experience. Hard materials like stone, metal, and glass can reflect sound and make a space feel echoey, which can hinder enjoyment and discussion. Soft furniture, including carpets, drapes, and upholstered chairs, can assist in absorbing sound and improve the acoustic environment. Additional options for lowering noise levels and improving the general comfort of the area include acoustic panels or wall treatments.

In contemporary dining areas, technology integration is becoming more and more crucial. Smart lighting, sound systems, and other tech upgrades can make dinner parties and family get-togethers more enjoyable for individuals who like to host. While smart lighting systems provide customizable lighting scenarios that can be altered with a smartphone or voice command, wireless speakers can play background music. Maintaining the dining area's appearance and functionality requires making sure technology is discreetly integrated and integrated.

The eating area gains a distinctive and significant dimension from cultural and individual touches. An environment that seems genuine and welcoming can be created by using components that honor cultural history, individual hobbies, or treasured experiences. This could be showcasing artwork, treasures from the family, or mementos from trips. These unique additions not only improve the room's aesthetic appeal but also foster a feeling of community and belonging.

A dining area that is both practical and pleasurable must prioritize comfort and ergonomics. It's crucial to make sure the table and chairs are at the right height for comfortable dining. Dining tables are normally 28 to 30 inches high, while chairs usually have an 18-inch seat height. To enhance comfort, consider the chair's depth and cushioning, as well as the distance between the table and chairs, which ought to provide effortless mobility and ample legroom.

Other crucial factors to think about include the eating area's accessibility and movement. The arrangement should make it simple to walk around and reach the table, storage spaces, and adjacent rooms. It is easier to serve and clean away food and dishes when there is a clear passage from the kitchen to the dining area. Additional seating alternatives, like benches or folding chairs, can accommodate more people during larger gatherings without taking up too much room.

The use of outdoor dining areas is growing in popularity as a great way to eat in the great outdoors. Choosing weatherproof equipment, suitable lighting, and taking the weather into account are all important when setting up an outside dining space. Strong and weatherproof, teak, aluminium, and synthetic wicker tables and chairs are a great choice. Evening dinners can have a mystical atmosphere created by outside lighting, such as solar-powered lamps, lanterns, and string lights. Making sure the outdoor eating area has enough shade and weather protection, like pergolas or umbrellas, improves its usability and comfort.

Special occasions and seasonal changes present chances to revamp and improve the eating area. For example, adding themed décor, unique table arrangements, and festive lighting to the dining area during holidays or festivities can make the space unforgettable and happy. Adding seasonal accents to the area, such as winter greenery, spring flowers, or fall leaves, keeps it lively and in step with the year's cycles.

Setting up a dining area with sustainability in mind is crucial. Making eco-friendly product and material choices—such as using recycled glass, organic fabrics, and wood from sustainably managed forests—supports environmental preservation and fosters a healthier home atmosphere. Purchasing sturdy, well-made furniture and décor also lessens the need for regular replacements, which supports a more sustainable way of living. Buying locally created furniture and décor items not only reduces the carbon footprint involved with long-distance shipping but also enhances the dining space's distinctiveness and authenticity by supporting local artisans and companies.

The dining area serves as a venue for celebration, interaction, and connection in addition to being a place for eating. An atmosphere that accentuates the dining experience and reflects individual style is created by thoughtful design and careful consideration of components like furniture, lighting, layout, decor, and practicality. The dining area can develop into a treasured and essential component of the house by putting comfort, style, and functionality first, creating loved meals and moments that will last for years.

In summary, designing a dining area requires a well-balanced combination of practicality, style, and individuality. A welcoming and cozy space is mostly determined by the furniture, lighting, arrangement, and décor choices made. An elegant dining area for hosting guests or a small, comfortable nook for family dinners, a well-designed dining area improves the dining experience and captures the essence of its owners' personalities and lifestyles. One may design a dining area that is not only lovely and practical but also a true representation of home and family by paying close attention to detail and considering elements like ergonomics, acoustics, sustainability, and cultural value.

The role of gratitude and mindfulness in eating

In order to maintain one's physical and emotional health, eating with awareness and thankfulness has garnered a lot of attention in recent years. These age-old customs, bolstered by contemporary science, provide significant advantages that go beyond simple nourishment. They make eating a holistic activity that nourishes the spirit, mind, and body. This section examines the relationship between eating with gratitude and mindfulness, emphasizing the historical background, physiological and psychological advantages, and real-world uses.

Both mindfulness—a concentrated attention on the present moment—and gratitude—an appreciation for what one has—have profound origins in a variety of philosophical and spiritual traditions. A fundamental component of Buddhism is mindfulness, which encourages people to give their experiences—including eating—their whole attention. Similar to this, many indigenous societies consider food to be a holy gift from the planet and emphasize being grateful for it. In contrast to the sometimes rushed and careless eating habits that are common in contemporary society, these behaviors promote a respectful and grateful relationship with food.

When eating mindfully, one must give complete attention to all aspects of the sensory experience, including the sight, texture, taste, and smell of the meal, as well as the physical feelings of fullness and hunger. Eating can become a rich and fulfilling experience with this technique instead of just being a mundane activity. People can improve their food enjoyment and strengthen their bond with their meals by taking their time and enjoying every bite. This raised awareness can help detect behavioral reasons for consuming food, including stress as well as monotony, in alongside fostering positive eating practices. When it comes to eating, being grateful means acknowledging and appreciating the resources and labor that go into growing and cooking food. This can involve giving gratitude to the chefs or family members who prepared the meal, the farmers who planted it, the laborers who gathered and delivered it, and the natural processes that made it all possible. These meal rituals can improve the entire dining experience by fostering a sense of interconnectedness and appreciation for the food on one's plate.

There is ample evidence supporting the psychological advantages of eating with awareness and thankfulness. It has been shown that by promoting calm and present-moment awareness, mindfulness training can reduce stress and anxiety. When it comes to eating, mindfulness can make people more aware of their bodies' signals of hunger and fullness, which lowers the risk of overindulging or emotional eating. A more balanced diet and a better relationship with food might result from this mindful eating style.

Conversely, gratitude has been connected to better mental and physical health. Regular expression of thankfulness can lessen the symptoms of anxiety and melancholy while raising emotions of contentment and happiness in life. Developing thankfulness for their meals can make people feel more satisfied and fulfilled, which can improve their mental health in general. Moreover, practicing thankfulness can help one adopt a more optimistic perspective on life by refocusing attention from what is lacking or desired to what is currently there and sufficient.

As important are the physiological advantages of attentive eating. According to research, mindful eating can facilitate better digestion by lowering stress levels and encouraging relaxation, both of which can impede the digestive process. People can minimize intestinal discomfort and improve nutrient absorption by eating slowly and carefully. A healthy weight can be encouraged, and overeating can be avoided by practicing mindfulness, which also promotes awareness of the body's signals of hunger and fullness.

Moreover, gratitude can improve one's physical well-being. People who consistently practice thankfulness tend to have higher immune systems and lower inflammatory levels, according to studies. This could be a result of gratitude's ability to lessen stress and lessen the negative consequences that long-term stress has on the body. Moreover, cultivating an attitude of gratitude can reinforce positive lifestyle decisions such as consuming correctly, exercising constantly, and getting restful sleep, all of whom enhance the quality of one's life.

There are several methods for integrating mindfulness and appreciation into eating habits. A typical practice is to start meals with a brief thank-you for the food or a moment of quiet. This custom, which is frequently observed in religious or cultural traditions, can serve to remind people of the value of thankfulness and assist in establishing a mindful atmosphere throughout the meal. Maintaining a thankfulness diary, where they record their daily blessings—including their meals—can be beneficial for certain individuals. This can strengthen the practice of thankfulness and increase its advantages.

Distraction-free dining is another useful strategy for mindful eating. People may concentrate entirely on the act of eating when they do not have to deal with interruptions from television, cell phones, or laptops while they eat. This can improve one's appreciation of food and increase awareness of one's own hunger and fullness cues. Slowing down, setting down utensils in between bites, and chewing every mouthful well can all help to improve digestion and foster mindfulness.

An essential component of mindful eating is engaging the senses. It is possible to improve the sensory experience and strengthen the bond with a meal by taking the time to enjoy the flavors, textures, and colors of food. Eating may become a joyful and engaging activity when one is aware of the flavors and textures in each bite. In addition to increasing meal satisfaction, this sensory engagement can lessen the propensity to overeat or seek out bad foods.

Observing the body's cues prior to, during, and after meals is another aspect of mindful eating. This entails identifying the difference between real hunger and emotional hunger, observing fullness sensations, and understanding the impact of various foods on mood and energy levels. People can make more thoughtful and informed dietary decisions that promote their health and well-being by tuning into these signals.

The broader context of food production and sustainability can also benefit from the application of gratitude and mindfulness while eating. More sustainable eating practices can be promoted by acknowledging the effects that food choices have on the environment and showing gratitude for the resources used in food production. Choosing foods that are obtained locally, organic, or plant-based can help reduce environmental impact. By becoming conscious of the sources and impacts of the food they eat, people can develop a higher regard for the assets of the world and contribute to the creation of a food system that is healthier for humanity.

Gratitude and mindful eating can improve shared experiences and build relationships in social and familial contexts. Family dinners offer a chance to practice thankfulness together, fostering a supportive and upbeat atmosphere. This might be as easy as passing along gratitude before a meal or talking about the history and health advantages of the food being shared. In addition to encouraging better eating habits and more solid interpersonal bonds, these activities can help families feel more united and appreciative of one another.

In social settings, practicing mindfulness can improve the quality of time spent together over meals and foster a more welcoming and attentive environment. People can strengthen their bonds and make enduring memories by living in the present and giving their all to the cuisine and company. Expressing gratitude to hosts, cooks, and other diners can improve the feeling of community and appreciation during social meals.

Children and young people can learn about the concepts of mindfulness and appreciation in the context of education. By introducing these activities, educators can encourage the formation of wholesome eating habits, including a positive connection with food from a young age. Exercises in mindful eating, gratitude journals, and conversations about the sustainability and source of food can cultivate an appreciation and mindfulness that transcends the dinner table.

Eating habits that incorporate mindfulness and gratitude can also be beneficial for workplace environments. Encouraging workers to take deliberate breaks and savor their meals without interruptions can improve output and overall well-being. Establishing areas for group meals and encouraging an attitude of thankfulness and admiration helps foster a happier and more encouraging work environment.

In the context of healthcare and therapeutic settings, the importance of mindfulness and thankfulness in eating is equally pertinent. Mindful eating techniques can be an important part of recovery and treatment for those with eating disorders or bad eating habits. People who practice mindfulness are better able to identify emotional triggers, change unhealthy coping methods, and become more conscious of their eating habits. By encouraging an optimistic and thankful perspective that can improve self-esteem and general well-being, gratitude can aid in the healing process.

Dietitians and nutritionists can include appreciation and mindfulness in their counseling and educational initiatives. Healthy eating practices and a better relationship with food can be supported by teaching clients to engage their senses, pay attention to their hunger and fullness cues, and express gratitude for their food. These methods offer a comprehensive approach to nutritional health and can be used in conjunction with conventional nutrition recommendations.

In conclusion, eating involves more than just the act of ingesting food; it also involves practicing mindfulness and thankfulness. These customs make eating a more fulfilling and comprehensive experience by providing significant psychological, physical, and social advantages. A conscious and appreciative relationship with food can improve one's physical health, increase one's enjoyment of meals, and create stronger bonds with oneself, other people, and the environment. A more balanced, fulfilling, and meaningful relationship with food can result from incorporating mindfulness and appreciation into eating habits. This can improve general well-being and create a more sustainable and connected environment.

Pre-meal rituals

Pre-meal rituals are customs followed before meals and have been a part of human civilization for ages. Although these customs differ greatly between countries and people, they frequently help the body and mind get ready for eating. They can be anything from religious prayers and thankfulness statements to everyday tasks like putting on the table and washing hands. Pre-meal rituals are important because they can increase social connections, cultivate awareness, improve dining experiences, and enhance general health and well-being. This section examines the several kinds of pre-meal rituals, their historical and cultural backgrounds, their advantages from a psychological and physical standpoint, and their applicability to modern society.

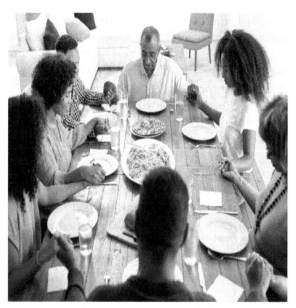

The custom of saying grace or reciting a prayer before dinner is among the most widespread pre-meal rituals. Numerous religious traditions, including Christianity, Judaism, Islam, Hinduism, and Buddhism, all practice this ceremony. Saying grace in Christianity typically entails giving thanks to God for the food and requesting His blessings. Before consuming certain foods, Jews say a particular set of blessings, called bracket, to express appreciation and acknowledgment of divine assistance. Reciting "Bismillah" (which means "In the name of Allah") before a meal is typical in Islam. This practice emphasizes attention and thankfulness. There are numerous pre-meal prayers and rituals in Buddhism and Hinduism that express gratitude and call out benefits. These religious customs sanctify the meal, strengthen the bonds of community among those who share it, and encourage appreciation and attentiveness in others.

Another typical pre-meal custom is expressing appreciation, whether via religious or secular channels. Enhancing the eating experience can be as simple as pausing to recognize and value the food, the labor of love that went into preparing it, and the people who made it possible. People are urged by this practice to appreciate the interdependence of the food chain and to live in the present. People can develop a positive outlook, as well as a sense of happiness and appreciation, by expressing thanks, all of which can enhance general well-being.

Pre-meal rituals are also greatly influenced by cultural traditions. Before dining, there are customs and practices that are followed in many cultures. For example, saying "Itadakimasu," which translates to "I humbly receive," before a meal is common in Japan. This expression expresses appreciation for the food and the labor of the people who cooked it. A comparable expression, "Jal meokgesseumnida," is used to show gratitude before to eating in Korea. These customs emphasize the cultural qualities of humility and respect in addition to the significance of appreciation.

Along with religious and cultural traditions, families and individuals engage in a range of beneficial pre-meal rituals. Hand washing before eating is a custom that encourages good hygiene and stops the transmission of germs. This custom has been followed for millennia in various countries and is especially significant in group dining settings. Another useful custom is setting the table, which entails positioning glasses, plates, napkins, and utensils in order to prepare the food. This can be a purposeful and thoughtful technique that contributes to a clean, comfortable dining area.

Pre-meal rituals for a lot of individuals usually entail some kind of thoughtful preparation, such as deep breathing, quiet time, or quick meditation. By assisting people in making the shift from the hectic pace of everyday life to a more concentrated and calm state, these techniques can improve their awareness and appreciation of the meal. Aside from mindful cooking, mindful preparation can also involve focusing on the visual, tactile, and olfactory components of food, which can enhance the enjoyment and appreciation of eating.

Pre-meal rituals that promote unity and connection are frequently a part of family customs and routines. Some families, for instance, might have a set sitting arrangement where each person has a specified spot at the table. Some might participate in a group activity like sharing their best moments of the day or talking about subjects they find interesting. These customs improve family ties and the dining experience by fostering a sense of structure and belonging.

It is commonly known that pre-meal routines provide psychological benefits. By encouraging serenity and relaxation, these activities can lower stress and anxiety. People can divert their attention from concerns and distractions by pausing and focusing on the here and now, which makes meals more tranquil and pleasurable. Pre-meal rituals have the potential to improve awareness, making people more aware of their hunger and fullness cues and encouraging them to eat healthily. Furthermore, expressing thanks before a meal might improve mood and general well-being by cultivating an optimistic outlook and lowering negative feelings.

As important are the physiological advantages of pre-meal routines. Hand washing and thoughtful meal preparation are two practices that can enhance general health and digestion. Hand washing before eating promotes better hygiene and health by limiting the transmission of germs and the danger of foodborne infections. Deep breathing exercises and quick meditations are examples of mindful preparation that can stimulate the parasympathetic nervous system, which enhances digestion and promotes calm. These rituals can improve nutrition absorption and lessen the discomfort associated with digestion by promoting relaxation.

Pre-meal customs are also very important for building community and a sense of social interaction. A basic human action that fosters interpersonal relationships and promotes social bonds is sharing a meal. Saying grace, expressing appreciation, or partaking in family customs are examples of pre-dinner rituals that can improve the sense of community and connection among those consuming the meal. These behaviors foster an environment that is encouraging and helpful, encouraging candid communication and admiration for one another.

Pre-meal rituals have value in modern living that goes beyond customary religious and cultural activities. Making time for pre-meal rituals can be a great way to slow down, think, and connect in a fast-paced and frequently stressful society. These customs can operate as a counterpoint to the rushed and preoccupied eating patterns prevalent in contemporary culture. Pre-meal rituals can improve overall quality of life and support social, emotional, and physical well-being by encouraging mindfulness and thankfulness.

Pre-meal ritual integration can take many different forms based on personal preferences and situational factors. It could involve more individualized routines for some people, while it might involve more traditional religious or cultural activities for others. Finding activities that align with one's values and wayof life is crucial, as is approaching them mindfully and intentionally.

Creating a regular pattern that fits in with everyday plans and activities is one useful way to implement pre-meal rituals. Simple rituals like hand washing, laying the table, and pausing for a moment of appreciation or quiet before meals can all be a part of this pattern. People can improve the dining experience by establishing a feeling of order and predictability through regular mealtime habits.

Incorporating mindfulness practices into routines before meals is an additional strategy. This can entail techniques like mindful eating observation, meditation, or deep breathing. By assisting people in making the shift from the hectic pace of everyday life to a more concentrated and at ease condition, these methods can improve their awareness and appreciation of the meal. The sensory experience of the food can be enhanced, and a deeper appreciation of the meal can be fostered by mindfully observing its colors, textures, and scents.

Establishing pre-meal rituals can help families spend more time together and in connection. This can entail doing things like saying thank you, sharing your favorite moments from the day, or carrying on family customs. These customs can improve family ties and foster a cheerful, encouraging dining atmosphere. Before a meal, for instance, some families might have a custom of joining hands and giving gratitude, while others might alternately take turns discussing something for which they are thankful. These customs improve the entire dining experience by fostering a sense of unity and appreciation.

Pre-meal rituals can strengthen the sense of togetherness and shared experience in social and communal contexts. This can entail customs like thanksgiving prayers, gatherings for communal activities, or group prayers. For instance, including pre-meal rituals can foster a welcoming environment in common dining areas like those found in companies, schools, or community centers. By encouraging a sense of community and support among one another, these activities can strengthen social ties and improve dining experiences in general.

Pre-meal rituals can be quite helpful in fostering both physical and mental well-being in therapeutic and medical settings. Pre-meal rituals can offer a regulated and encouraging framework for those with eating disorders or bad eating habits to build healthier connections with food. These techniques help improve mindfulness, lessen tension and anxiety, and encourage healthy eating habits. People can improve their eating habits and general well-being by increasing their awareness of their feelings of fullness and hunger cues by engaging in activities that foster mindfulness, such as respiration or meditation, before meals.

In school settings, teaching young people pre-meal rituals can support the early development of nutritious eating patterns and an enjoyable connection with food. Exercises in mindful eating, gratitude journals, and conversations about the sustainability and source of food can cultivate an appreciation and mindfulness that transcends the dinner table. Teachers can assist children in forming lifelong habits that support their physical, mental, and social well-being by implementing these practices at a young age.

In summary, pre-meal rituals have many psychological, physical, and social advantages and are an essential component of human culture and experience. These rituals —religious, cultural, or utilitarian—help the body and mind become ready for eating by encouraging mindfulness, appreciation, and community. Pre-meal rituals can be incorporated into daily life to improve the eating experience overall, support mental and physical health, and fortify social ties. Pre-meal rituals can offer a critical opportunity to calm down, think, and connect in a world where things move quickly and are sometimes stressful. This can lead to a more meaningful, balanced, and enjoyable relationship with food.

The importance of eating carefully

In a world where time is passing by at an ever-increasing rate, eating deliberately and appreciating every bite has become a crucial but frequently neglected habit. Fast food, multitasking, and hectic schedules have made it common for people to speed through meals and not enjoy the process of eating. This section explores the several benefits of eating slowly and deliberately, emphasizing the advantages for the state of one's mind and body along with social interactions. People can improve their general quality of life by comprehending and adopting this mindful eating style.

Eating slowly improves digestion, which is one of its main advantages. When food is chewed and combined with saliva, which includes digestive enzymes, the process of digestion starts in the mouth. By fully chewing food, these enzymes can start to break down fats and carbs, which facilitates faster nutrient absorption and further digestion in the stomach and intestines. Larger, undigested food particles enter the stomach when food is swallowed too rapidly and is not adequately chewed, which can cause indigestion, bloating, and pain. People can lessen their risk of developing gastrointestinal problems and enhance their digestive health by taking the time to chew their meals thoroughly.

Additionally, eating slowly helps the body better control signals of hunger and fullness. After around twenty minutes, the stomach sends signals to the brain indicating fullness. When people eat rapidly, they can take in more food than their bodies require before feeling satisfied, which could result in overindulgence and weight gain. However, eating slowly allows the body enough time to interpret these cues, assisting people in identifying when they are full and lowering the likelihood of overindulging. You can help yourself maintain a normal weight and prevent obesity-related health problems, including coronary artery disease, diabetes, and metabolic syndrome, by practicing mindful eating.

Eating deliberately and appreciating each bite has numerous health benefits for the body, but it can also greatly improve psychological well-being. It has been demonstrated that mindful eating, which is being fully present and conscious of the eating experience, lowers stress and enhances mental health. Focusing on the flavor, texture, and aroma of food, as well as the tactile experiences of chewing and swallowing, are all encouraged by mindful eating. This concentration has the potential to have a grounding and relaxing impact, which can lessen anxiety and encourage relaxation. Those who transform mealtimes into mindful periods can develop a stronger sense of serenity and well-being.

Moreover, mindful eating can support people in creating a more positive connection with food. Emotional eating is a common problem among those who use food as a coping mechanism for unpleasant feelings like stress, melancholy, or boredom. This may result in a vicious cycle of guilt and humiliation, as well as unhealthy eating habits. People can learn more about their emotional triggers and create more positive coping mechanisms by eating slowly and deliberately. Those who practice mindful eating are better able to recognize and react to their body's true signals of completeness and hunger, as opposed to utilizing food as a substitute for frightened and crutch. It does this by promoting a non-judgmental awareness of one's thoughts and feelings.

Eating carefully and appreciating every meal can also improve social interactions, which is another significant component of the dining experience. Mealtime gatherings with loved ones, friends, and coworkers offer chances for conversation, bonding, and social contact. People who eat quickly lose out on the opportunity to socialize and enjoy the communal component of eating. Relationships can be strengthened, and significant social experiences can be created by taking the time to eat leisurely and have meaningful conversations. Eating at a leisurely pace is a sign of respect for the social customs of family and community that are deeply ingrained in many cultures.

Eating slowly can improve food perception and enjoyment in addition to promoting social bonds. Food provides joy and satisfaction in addition to being a source of nutrition. Eating at a leisurely pace enhances the dining experience by allowing people to completely appreciate the flavors, textures, and fragrances of their food. Meals may become more satisfying and pleasurable as a result of this increased sensory awareness and contentment. People can develop a deeper respect for the art of cooking and the work that goes into creating a meal by taking the time to enjoy the culinary experience.

It's also important to consider the cultural and historical significance of eating slowly. The value of unhurried meals is strongly emphasized in many traditional societies. For instance, meals are frequently viewed as prolonged social gatherings where family and friends get together to enjoy food, wine, and conversation over a number of hours in Mediterranean nations like Greece and Italy. This eating style reflects a strong cultural value placed on the social and sensory components of food. In a similar vein, the Japanese custom of "ichiju-sansai" (one soup, three sides) promotes a mindful and balanced style of eating in which each course is carefully considered and enjoyed.

The fast-paced, convenience-driven eating style that has grown commonplace in many areas of the world has given rise to the slow food movement in modern civilization. The slow food movement promotes attentive, sustainable, and traditional eating habits. It highlights how important it is to set aside time to prepare and savor meals created with premium, locally produced products. The slow food movement supports eating slowly and appreciating every mouthful by advancing the ideals of sustainability, community, and enjoyment of food.

Even though eating slowly has many advantages, many people find it difficult to incorporate this habit into their daily lives. Meals should be enjoyed slowly because work, family, and other obligations often take up a lot of time. Furthermore, the widespread practice of multitasking, in which people eat while using electronic devices, watching TV, or working, might take away from the focused eating experience. Nonetheless, there are a number of methods that people can employ to make thoughtful and slow eating a regular part of their lives.

Establishing a focused dining area with few distractions is one useful tactic. This may entail designating a certain time and location for meals that are unaffected by distractions like electronics. The whole meal experience can be improved, and mindful eating can be promoted by designing a serene and welcoming dining area. Furthermore, cultivating appreciation before meals—for example, by pausing to acknowledge the food and the people who produced it—can create a happy and thoughtful atmosphere for the meal.

Concentrating on the eating experience as a sensory experience is another tactic. This can entail observing the food's flavors, textures, and colors as well as the actual physical experiences of chewing and swallowing. Using all of your senses can help you enjoy your meals more and be more mindful while eating. Furthermore, chewing carefully and taking smaller bits can aid in enhancing digestion and slowing down the eating process.

Including mindful eating techniques in group meals can also be beneficial. Eating meals together gives people a chance to catch up over discussion and enjoy the food. People can fortify their social ties and forge deep connections by setting aside time to savor the company of others and the gastronomic experience. Cooking and meal preparation with loved ones or friends can also increase one's appreciation for the food and the work that goes into its preparation.

In conclusion, there are many advantages to eating slowly and appreciating every meal for your physical and mental health as well as your social life. Eating slowly can enhance general health and well-being by creating a healthier connection with food, managing hunger and satiety signals, and improving digestion. Mindful eating has also been shown to lower stress, improve food satisfaction, and strengthen social bonds. Incorporating slow and mindful eating techniques into daily routines can improve overall quality of life and foster a greater appreciation for the act of eating, even in the face of modern life's obstacles. People who adopt this mindful eating style might develop a closer bond with their food, their bodies, and the environment.

Gentle detox recipes and practices

Many individuals look to detoxification as a means of revitalizing their bodies and brains in the midst of the hectic pace of modern life. The process of removing toxins from the body to improve general health and well-being is known as detoxification or detox. While there are many different detoxification techniques, such as fasting and tight diets, a more moderate strategy that includes whole foods and focused activities is frequently more long-term advantageous. The idea of a gentle detox is examined in this section, with an emphasis on activities and recipes that encourage the body's natural detoxification processes without placing undue strain or limits on the body.

Natural body processes include detoxification, which is mostly handled by the digestive tract, lungs, liver, kidneys, and skin. Toxins and waste materials are continuously filtered and removed by these organs. However, stress, processed foods, and pollution exposure can tax these systems, so it's good to support them with dietary and lifestyle choices. The goal of gentle detoxification techniques is to support the body's natural detoxification processes while minimizing toxic intake and nourishing the body.

Hydration is one of the main components of a mild detox. Water is necessary for all body functions, including detoxification, to operate correctly. It facilitates the movement of nutrients, the elimination of waste, and the preservation of biological processes. Throughout the day, consuming enough water can aid in the removal of toxins and maintain renal function. Water that has been infused, like that with lemon, cucumber, or mint segments, can improve hydration and offer further detoxification advantages. Lemon, for example, has antioxidants and vitamin C that assist the immune system and liver function.

Including whole, nutrient-dense foods in your diet is another essential element of a mild detox. Fresh produce is particularly healthful because it is high in fiber, antioxidants, trace elements, antioxidants, and other nutrients. These nutrients support the human body's detoxification processes and improve overall wellness. Leafy greens like greens such as kale, spinach, and arugula contain chlorophyll, which helps cleanse the liver and blood. Cruciferous vegetables, such as florets and Brussels sprouts, have compounds that help liver enzyme activity and enhance detoxification.

A smoothie made with greens is an easy and powerful detox dish. Green smoothies are nutrient-dense and easily digested since they combine a range of greens with fruits and a liquid basis. A simple dish might have half a diced cucumber, a green fruit, a cup of kale, a handful of spinach, a slice of Meyer ginger, which is also and a cup of the water from the coconuts. When these components are blended, a revitalizing beverage that supports detoxification with vitamins, minerals, and antioxidants is produced. To increase fiber content and support digestion and toxin removal, try adding a spoonful of chia or flaxseeds.

Fiber is essential for detoxification, especially in terms of gut health. It facilitates regular bowel movements and guarantees effective waste removal. Rich in dietary fiber are nuts, seeds, whole grain products, fruits, and vegetables. For instance, a healthy breakfast that aids in detoxification and digestion can be made with a bowl of oats garnished with fresh berries, flaxseeds, and honey. Furthermore, adding legumes to meals—such as beans, lentils, and chickpeas—can supply soluble and insoluble fiber, which supports regularity and intestinal health.

Another mild detox method that's simple to include in everyday life is herbal tea. Certain herbs assist liver function, improve digestion, and lower inflammation through their cleansing qualities. For example, dandelion root tea is well-known for supporting liver detoxification and stimulating bile synthesis. Similarly, silymarin, a substance that shields and encourages liver cell regeneration, is present in milk thistle tea. It can be a calming routine to sip a cup of herbal tea in the morning or evening, which supports relaxation and detoxification.

Gentle detoxification methods frequently involve mindful activities that lower stress and enhance general well-being in addition to food choices. The body's capacity to detoxify can be significantly impacted by stress, as prolonged stress can exacerbate liver damage and raise free radical generation. Deep breathing exercises, yoga, and meditation are examples of mindfulness practices that can lower stress and aid in detoxification. For example, practicing yoga's forward bends and twists, which excite the gastrointestinal tract, can help facilitate better digestion and the elimination of toxins.

Meditation is a useful mindful exercise that eases tension and promotes mental calmness. Daily meditation, even for just a short while, can significantly improve well-being. The relaxation response can be strengthened, and the body's natural detoxification processes can be supported via guided meditations that emphasize deep breathing and body awareness. Regular exercise, such as swimming, dancing, or walking, can also improve lymphatic drainage, stimulate circulation, and aid in the body's natural process of sweating out toxins.

Dry brushing is a mild detoxification technique that promotes lymphatic drainage and skin health. The largest organ in the body, the skin, is essential to detoxification. Using a natural bristle tool to gently exfoliate the skin may help flush away dead skin cells and pollutants while also boosting local blood flow. Before having a shower, you can do this circular exercise, beginning at the ankles and gradually working your way up. Dry brushing encourages smooth, healthy skin in addition to detoxifying.

Including fermented foods in the diet is another advantageous detoxification technique. Probiotics, found in fermented foods like kimchi, kefir, yogurt, and sauerkraut, help intestinal health and improve the body's detoxification capabilities. Immune system performance, nutrition absorption, and digestion are all significantly impacted by the gut flora. Fermented foods can aid in detoxification and general health by maintaining a balanced population of good bacteria in the gut. For example, eating a modest amount of sauerkraut or kimchi with meals helps flavor the diet and supply probiotics.

Time-restricted eating or intermittent fasting may also be part of a mild detox program. These methods entail restricting the amount of time one can consume each day so that fasting intervals can be used by the body to recuperate and repair. A biological mechanism called autophagy, which eliminates damaged cells and encourages regeneration, can be improved by intermittent fasting. This procedure can enhance general health and aid in cellular detoxification. The 16/8 method is a popular strategy in which people fast for 16 hours and eat within an 8-hour timeframe. You can do this by not eating breakfast, eating your first meal at midday, and continuing to eat until eight o'clock at night.

A healthy sleep schedule is another crucial element of a gradual detox. The body goes through several restorative processes when you sleep, one of which is the lymphatic system clearing waste products out of the brain. Inadequate slumber can hinder these mechanisms and lead to the build-up of poisons. The body can detoxify more effectively if a regular sleep schedule and a peaceful sleep environment are established. This could entail minimizing screen time before bed, engaging in relaxation exercises, and making sure that the bedroom is quiet, dark, and cozy.

Including a range of foods high in nutrients in the diet can help promote a more gradual detoxification process. Antioxidant-rich foods like dark chocolate, nuts, seeds, and berries aid in the neutralization of free radicals and shield cells from harm. Spices like turmeric, which have anti-inflammatory and antioxidant qualities, can be used in food or drunk as golden milk. Golden milk is a calming beverage that promotes detoxification and general wellness. It is produced by boiling milk (or a plant-based substitute) with turmeric, black pepper, and a small amount of honey.

Herbs and leafy greens are also essential for detoxification. Add mint, parsley, and cilantro to salads, juices, and juices to enhance cleansing. In particular, cilantro is widely known for its ability to bind to toxic substances and support the body's natural removal of them. Tossed greens, shredded carrots, cucumber, avocado, a few fresh herbs, and a lemon-tahini dressing might make up a basic detox salad. This concoction offers vitamins, minerals, good fats, and substances that aid in detoxification.

Another well-liked moderate detox method is juicing. Vitamins, minerals, and antioxidants are concentrated in pure fruit and vegetable juices. Juicing might be especially beneficial for people who have trouble eating enough fruits and vegetables. Carrots, apples, celery, ginger, and a squeeze of lemon are possible ingredients in a simple juice preparation. This blend is not only immune-boosting and refreshing, but it also helps with digestion and liver function. To guarantee enough fiber consumption, it's crucial to mix juicing with entire foods.

Another delectable approach to include foods that aid in detoxification in the diet is through smoothie bowls. You may alter these nutrient-dense bowls by adding different fruits, veggies, nuts, seeds, and superfoods. A base of blended spinach, banana, pineapple, and almond milk may be the basis of a detox smoothie bowl. Chia seeds, hemp hearts, goji berries, and almond butter drizzle over the top. Fiber, protein, good fats, and antioxidants are all included in this combo to help with detoxification and general wellness.

A mild detoxification can be supported by certain supplements in addition to food and lifestyle changes. For instance, milk thistle is a well-known liver tonic that promotes liver regeneration and function. Consuming a supplement containing milk thistle can improve the liver's capacity to break down and remove poisons. Probiotics, which improve intestinal health, and omega-3 fatty acids, which lower inflammation and promote cellular health, are two more advantageous supplements. It's imperative to see a healthcare professional before starting any new supplements to ensure they meet your needs.

Lastly, developing a durable and well-balanced detoxification strategy is essential. Restrictive diets and extreme detoxification techniques can be stressful and ineffective, resulting in nutrient shortages and other health problems. Keeping hydrated, feeding the body complete foods, and adding mindful practices that promote general well-being are the main components of a gentle detox. This strategy not only encourages long-term health and vitality but is also more sustainable.

To sum up, mild detoxification techniques and recipes provide an all-encompassing and long-lasting approach to bolster the body's innate detoxification mechanisms. Enhancing their overall health and wellness can be achieved through increasing nutrient-dense food intake, maintaining adequate hydration, practicing mindfulness, and engaging in regular exercise. Lightweight detoxification techniques, like drinking herbal teas, consuming fermented foods, making green smoothies, and dry brushing, can assist in the process without putting too much pressure on the body. People can improve their general health, their quality of life, and their connection to their bodies by adopting a balanced and thoughtful approach to detoxification.

CONCLUSION

Upon finishing "Ayurvedic Kitchen Secrets: Balancing Body and Mind Through Ancient Recipes," you will have had a profound and enlightening voyage into the core of Ayurvedic knowledge. You now have a deep grasp of how traditional eating practices may balance and revitalize your body and mind thanks to this book. You are strengthening your inner well-being and nurturing your physical self at the same time when you include these recipes and concepts into your everyday life.

The variety of recipes included in this book shows that Ayurveda is not a set system but rather an adaptable manual that can be unique to address the specific needs and preferences of each individual. Every dish serves as a reminder of the significant influence mindful eating can have on your health, whether you have found solace in the warming spices, harmony in the dosha-specific meals, or delight in the seasonal foods.

"Ayurvedic Kitchen Secrets" gives you the information and skills you need to make decisions that are in line with your particular constitution. It gives you the ability to cook scrumptious and healthful meals, encouraging a way of life that values prevention, balance, and overall well-being. I wish you well as you continue to study and implement these Ayurvedic principles. May your kitchen become a healing space where each meal you cook is a step closer to greater harmony and energy.

Accept the knowledge of Ayurveda and allow it to lead you to a happy, healthy life.

Thank you for buying and reading/listening to our book. If you found this book useful/helpful please take a few minutes and leave a review on the platform where you purchased our book. Your feedback matters greatly to us.

Printed in the USA
CPSIA information can be obtained
at www.ICGtesting.com
CBHW060344070824
12784CB00054B/763